the**facts**

Heart disease

ADRIAN CHENZBRAUN, MD, FRCP, FESC
Consultant Cardiologist
The Royal Liverpool University Hospital
The Liverpool Heart and Chest Hospital

OXFORD
UNIVERSITY PRESS

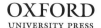

OXFORD
UNIVERSITY PRESS

Great Clarendon Street, Oxford OX2 6DP

Oxford University Press is a department of the University of Oxford.
It furthers the University's objective of excellence in research, scholarship,
and education by publishing worldwide in

Oxford New York

Athens Auckland Bangkok Bogotá Buenos Aires Calcutta
Cape-Town Chennai Dar-es-Salaam Delhi Florence Hong-Kong Istanbul
Karachi Kuala-Lumpur Madrid Melbourne Mexico-City Mumbai
Nairobi Paris São-Paulo Singapore Taipei Tokyo Toronto Warsaw

with associated companies in Berlin Ibadan

Oxford is a registered trade mark of Oxford University Press
in the UK and in certain other countries

Published in the United States
by Oxford University Press Inc., New York

© Oxford University Press, 2010

British Library Cataloguing in Publication Data

Data available

Library of Congress Cataloguing in Publication Data

ISBN 978-0-19-9582815

10 9 8 7 6 5 4 3 2 1

Foreword

It has become rather common practice to open a foreword to a publication of this ranking, or indeed any on the matter of heart disease, with a reminder to you, the reader, that more than 300,000 people in the UK have a heart attack each year and furthermore, that one in four of us will die of heart disease. So how do I, no less keen than all my health professional friends and colleagues, in any new way raise the clarion call to a higher level and urge us to seek out change in what appears to be a society that still remains reluctant to listen to the best advice?

The fact is that we can all positively individually influence our health in so many ways, from the food we eat and the exercize we take, to the partnerships we must build with our clinicians and general practitioners. Being 'doctored' should not remove the elements of control for either partner, but instead bring joint control to the surgery. This joint involvement should thus begin the process of our return to the 'art of doctoring'.

Risk factor management is now an essential skill and is, or should be, more about day-to-day front line care. Advances in that care are with us today and make it possible for physicians to modify the course of disease in many new and innovative ways. So while this publication is aimed broadly at the public, those physicians and other health professionals interested in the prevention, diagnosis, and treatment of cardiovascular disease will also be reminded and mindful of the role they so importantly play. For instance, the NICE FH (Familial Hypercholesterolaemia) Guidelines published in August 2008 in the UK recommended the screening of family members diagnosed with FH. The importance of such screening cannot be underemphasized as it allows for the diagnosis, identification and treatment of those affected and thus their risk reduction of developing CHD. So there is many a reason for the well-informed and eager-to-learn patient to take note of the pages herein, so rich in state-of-the-art resources, clearly defined referral sections—all presented in a well laid out format.

I am sure that this publication will ably help in those endeavours, for *Heart Disease: The Facts* offers that perfect practical guide on the rationale for decision-making in clinical practice between those in primary care and the patient who has today truly begun to understand the need for their presence—not as an outsider to discussion and decision—but as one who is present and thus a benefitting participant in a new working partnership.

Michael Livingston

Director, InterChol—The International Cholesterol Foundation

Preface

Why this book?

For the last 100 years, we have been witnessing a tremendous increase in the frequency of diseases of the heart and blood vessels (cardiovascular diseases). There are many reasons for this, several of which are complex, but they have to do with profound economic, social, and demographic changes, mainly industrialization, urbanization, low levels of physical activity (sedentarism), and the increased availability of fat- and calorie-rich food. Around the 1970s, cardiovascular mortality began to decrease in the Western world because of improved health consciousness and better medical care, but nevertheless cardiovascular diseases still account for about half of all deaths in the developed countries and 25% of deaths in the developing world (compared with only 10% worldwide at the beginning of the 20th century).

As a result of increased life expectancy and improved early detection, the number of individuals with either manifest cardiovascular disease, or those at risk of developing it, is continuously growing. With that comes the need for available information on this ailment and the ways to fight it.

Who should read this book and what will you find in it?

This book is directed at the public at large, both those with and those without heart disease. It intends to be a practical guide to help you understand common cardiac conditions and frequently used medical terms and concepts. The book opens with a general presentation of the structure and function of the cardiovascular system, followed by chapters dealing with specific cardiac diseases. The chapters begin with a summary of the key points and include frequently asked questions that are likely to be of interest to a cardiac patient. These questions have been compiled by the author using experience accumulated through 20 years of interaction with patients and colleagues both in hospital and in outpatient clinics. Both the usual concerns and anxieties of a newly diagnosed cardiac patient and the more 'professional' questions of inquisitive and 'seasoned' individuals are addressed. A guide to the main cardiac medications can be found at the end of the book.

Although targeted mainly at cardiac patients, this book will also be useful for paramedics, specialist nurses, support groups, GPs, and all those involved in treating heart patients in the community.

How to use this book?

The book begins with the structure and functioning of the heart, followed by a description of specific cardiac conditions, and ends with a presentation of commonly used cardiovascular drugs and devices. However, it does not have to be read 'cover to cover'. To facilitate this approach, reference is made when the same issue is discussed in more than one chapter. Plain language and lay terms are used throughout the book, but medical terms are mentioned as well, when appropriate, and a glossary is provided.

Contents

Section 3
Treatment

Symbols and abbreviations

≥	greater than or equal to
≤	less than or equal to
ACE	angiotensin-converting enzyme
AF	atrial fibrillation
AFl	atrial flutter
AHT	arterial hypertension
AP	angina pectoris
AR	aortic regurgitation
ARB	angiotensin receptor blocker
ARVC	arrhythmogenic right ventricular cardiomyopathy
AS	aortic stenosis
ASD	atrial septal defect
AVB	atrioventricular block
BAV	bicuspid aortic valve
BMI	body mass index
BMS	bare metal stent
BP	blood pressure
CABG	coronary artery bypass graft
CAD	coronary artery disease
CCU	coronary care unit
CHD	congenital heart disease
CHF	congestive heart failure
CT	computed tomography
DCC	direct current cardioversion

DCMP	dilated cardiomyopathy
DES	drug-eluting stent
DM	diabetes mellitus
ECG	electrocardiogram
EF	ejection fraction
GP	general practitioner
GTN	nitroglycerin
HCM	hypertrophic cardiomyopathy
HDL	high-density lipoprotein
ICD	implantable cardioverter–defibrillator
IE	infective endocarditis
IHD	ischaemic heart disease
INR	international normalized ratio
LAD	left anterior descending artery
LCX	left circumflex artery
LDL	low-density lipoprotein
LMCA	left main coronary artery
LQTS	long-QT syndrome
LVAD	left ventricular assist devices
mcg	microgram
Met	metabolic unit
MI	myocardial infarction
mmHg	millimetres of mercury
MR	mitral regurgitation
MRI	magnetic resonance imaging
MS	mitral stenosis
MVP	mitral valve prolapse
NSAID	non-steroidal anti-inflammatory drug
NSTEMI	non-ST-elevation myocardial infarction
PCI	percutaneous coronary intervention
PDA	patent ductus arteriosus
PFO	patent foramen ovale

POTS	postural tachycardia syndrome
PPCMP	peripartum cardiomyopathy
PS	pulmonary stenosis
PSVT	paroxysmal supraventricular tachycardia
PTCA	percutaneous transluminal coronary angioplasty
RCA	right coronary artery
SCD	sudden cardiac death
SOB	shortness of breath
STEMI	ST-elevation myocardial infarction
STK	streptokinase
TOE	transoesophageal echocardiography
TTE	transthoracic echocardiography
VF	ventricular fibrillation
VSD	ventricular septal defect
VT	ventricular tachycardia

Section 1

The facts about heart disease

1

How does the cardiovascular system work?

🔁 Key Points

- The circulatory or cardiovascular system comprises the heart, a muscle which acts as a pump to move blood around the body, and the blood vessels, which connect the heart with the whole body.

- When blood passes through the lungs, it is enriched with oxygen, which is delivered to the tissues, from which carbon dioxide (CO_2) is brought back to lungs to be eliminated into the atmosphere.

- In order to perform this action the heart normally pumps, or beats, 60–90 times a minute. This is our heart rate that can be recorded as the pulse.

- The heart muscle, like any other tissue in the body, needs its own blood supply. This is provided by the two coronary arteries that arise from the aorta and course across the heart surface. The narrowing of these arteries or their branches can be responsible for heart disease.

The cardiovascular system ensures that the blood is moved around the body in a closed circuit (Fig. 1.1) to deliver oxygen, hormones, and other biologically active substances to all organs and to remove the products of cell metabolism that are no longer needed. The vessels taking the oxygen-enriched blood from the heart are called arteries, and the ones bringing the blood back from the organs are called veins. At their ends, the arteries and the veins become very small (arterioles and venules) and are connected by a meshwork of tiny vessels (capillaries) that supply blood directly to organs and tissues.

The oxygenated blood leaves the left ventricle of the heart to be distributed by the aorta and its branches to all the body organs and tissues. The blood is then returned to the right side of the heart through venous branches that converge

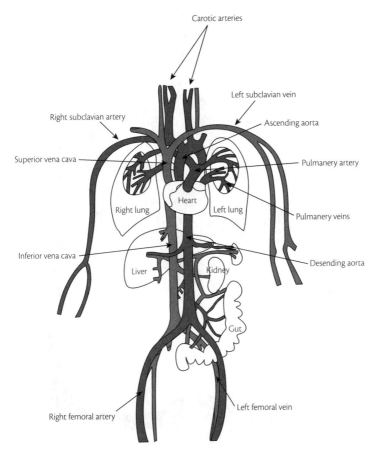

Figure 1.1 Schematic representation of the circulatory system (arteries in dark grey, veins in light grey). The aorta originates from the left ventricle, has an upward segment (ascending aorta) that provides the main arteries for the head (carotid arteries), and then curves downwards (descending aorta) to provide the subclavian arteries for the upper limbs, arteries for various chest and abdominal organs, and the femoral arteries for the lower limbs. The veins collecting the venous blood from the head and upper arms conflate into the superior vena cava while those collecting the blood from the rest of the body conflate into the inferior vena cava.

into the two venae cavae. The right ventricle pumps the returning blood through the pulmonary artery to the lungs, where CO_2 is eliminated and the blood is re-enriched with oxygen. From the lungs the blood is directed through the pulmonary veins to the left side of the heart to be pumped through the aorta again (Fig. 1.2).

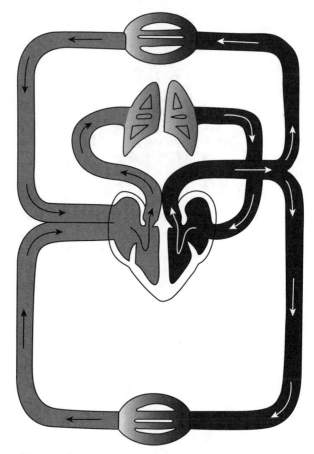

Figure 1.2 Schematic drawing of the continuous heart-driven flow motion that takes oxygenated blood to tissues and brings it back to lungs for re-oxygenation: light grey, venous blood; dark grey, oxygenated arterial blood. For details of the intra-cardiac blood flow, see text and Figure 1.3.

The pump action of the heart

To ensure this continuous flow, the heart is built as a sophisticated pump. It contains four cavities (two ventricles and two atria), grouped in two atrium–ventricle pairs, one on the left side and one on the right side. A system of four valves ensures the unidirectional flow of the blood within the heart: the tricuspid valve allows the filling of the right ventricle from the right atrium, the pulmonic valve controls the emptying of the right ventricle through the pulmonary artery, the mitral valve regulates the filling of the left ventricle from the left atrium and, finally, the aortic valve controls the ejection of oxygenated blood from the left ventricle into the aorta (Fig. 1.3).

The build of the heart

The heart walls have a three-layered structure:

- a thin inner layer (endocardium), from which the valvular structures arise
- a thick muscular mid-layer (myocardium), responsible for heart contraction
- a thin external layer (pericardium) that envelops the heart.

The mechanical activity of the heart is a regular and timely succession of contraction and expansion of heart cavities, responsible for the heart pumping activity which, in an adult at rest, results in the circulation of about 7000 litres over 24 hours. This impressive mechanical activity is controlled by electrical impulses that normally originate in the upper part of the right atrium and propagate within the heart to stimulate the muscular contraction (Fig. 1.4). Finally, like any other organ, the heart itself needs its own blood supply which is provided by the coronary arteries (Fig. 1.5). The two major coronary trunks originate in the proximal aortic root, just above the aortic valve, and then curve around the heart and provide branches through which oxygenated blood is delivered to the myocardium. Obstructions in the coronary tree are responsible for angina and heart attacks.

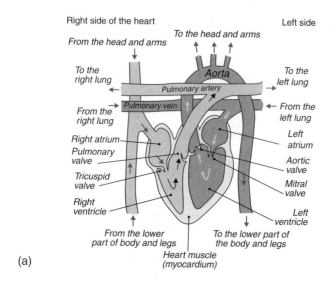

(a)

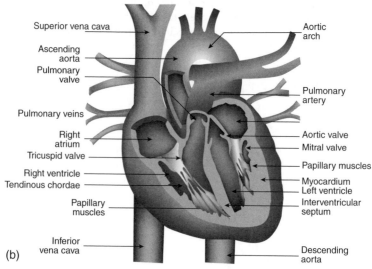

(b)

Figure 1.3 Schematic representation of (a) the direction of the intra-cardiac flow as controlled by the heart valves and (b) the heart internal build: light grey, venous blood; dark grey, oxygenated arterial blood.

(Reproduced with kind permission of the British Heart Foundation, the copyright owner)

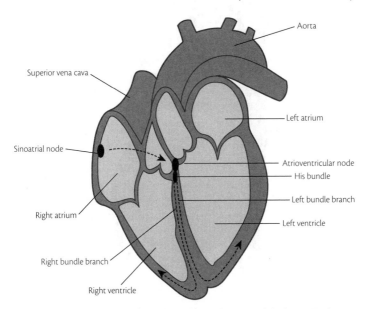

Figure 1.4 Schematic representation of the electrical system of the heart. Cardiac impulses are generated by the sinoatrial node, a cluster of cells located in the right atrium, and propagate to another group of cells, the atrioventricular node. The electrical impulse is briefly delayed at this level, so that ventricular contraction will not occur at the same time as atrial contraction, and it further advances through the His bundle and its two right and left branches until all the heart muscle is activated and ventricular contraction is initiated.

(Reproduced with kind permission of the British Heart Foundation, the copyright owner)

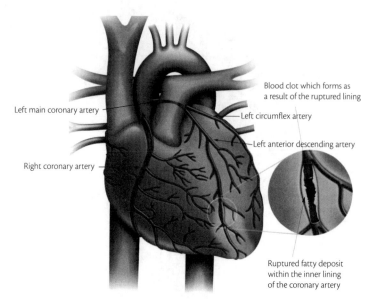

Blood clot which forms as
a result of the ruptured lining

Left main coronary artery

Left circumflex artery

Left anterior descending artery

Right coronary artery

Ruptured fatty deposit
within the inner lining
of the coronary artery

Figure 1.5 External aspect of the heart and course of the coronary arteries. The right coronary artery (RCA) supplies mainly the right ventricle and the inferior wall of the left ventricle. The left main coronary artery (LMCA), divides itself into the left anterior descending artery (LAD) that supplies mainly the anterior wall of the heart and its apex and the left circumflex artery (LCX) that supplies mainly the lateral wall of the heart.

(Reproduced with the kind permission of the British Heart Foundation, the copyright owner)

2

What are the symptoms of heart disease?

> ## ➔ Key Points
>
> - Chest pain, palpitations, shortness of breath, fainting, and leg swelling are associated with heart disease.
> - Chest pain is the central symptom in angina and heart attack. Frequently, its features are typical enough to allow a presumptive diagnosis even before more specialized tests are performed.
> - Palpitations are a very common cardiac symptom, and are usually associated with rhythm disturbances. Although palpitations may be perceived as very unpleasant and cause anxiety, they are not necessarily associated with a significant heart disease.
> - Shortness of breath may be the main cardiac symptom in some patients, but its subjective nature and presence in many other conditions as well may render the diagnosis difficult.

Chest pain

Chest pain is a very frequent complaint encountered in many conditions from a tense chest muscle to heart disease. It is the defining symptom of angina and heart attack and, as such, it has a serious emotional impact and raises concerns not associated with pains in other body areas. As a rule, the diagnosis must rest with your physician, and sometimes the decision is difficult even for experienced cardiologists. However, the following characteristics of the pain can help you decide whether it might be anginal or not (Table 2.1). Also, as a general rule, the younger you are (less than 50 years for women and less than 40 years for men), the lower the chances are that your pain is cardiac in origin.

One last word of caution: The guidelines above relate to ischaemic pain, i.e. pain related to narrowing of the arteries of the heart, as in heart attack or angina. There are some other instances of chest pain possibly related to the heart, like inflammation of the tissue layer covering the heart (the pericard). Although less common, this diagnosis should be kept in mind if sharp severe pain, related to

Table 2.1 Usual features of anginal pain compared with other chest-related pains

	Low chance the pain is cardiac	High chance the pain is cardiac: seek medical attention!
Pain characteristics	Short-lived stabbing sharp pain	Pressure, heaviness, burning, ill-defined discomfort, excruciating pain
Pain location	Right chest, 'point' area 'over the heart', easy to define area. Does not irradiate	Mid-chest, difficult to delineate area. May extend to neck, jaw, shoulders, back
Pain duration	A few seconds. Hours of constant pain	A few minutes up to a few hours
Associated complaints	No	Yes
Occurrence	Unpredictable, more at rest than during activities	When walking/climbing stairs, after meals, when exposed to cold

breathing, appears during or after some 'flu-like disease'. As a rule, any unusual chest pain occurring together with other worrying symptoms such as shortness of breath, fatigue, nausea, dizziness, or sweating should prompt you to seek medical attention.

Palpitations/irregular pulse

Palpitations are a common complaint which frequently bring people to consult a cardiologist. The description may vary: 'strong heart beat', 'rapid pulse', or 'my heart skips a beat'. In some cases there is absolutely no abnormality behind these complaints; some individuals just perceive normal changes in their heart rhythm in an unpleasant way. In other cases, there is a real disturbance in the heart rhythm, although it does not necessarily mean that disease is present. Treatment is available, but in many cases it is unnecessary. As a rule of thumb, the occurrence of rare, well-tolerated, and isolated palpitations in a young person without any evidence of heart disease is a benign symptom that does not warrant treatment or investigation. Again, the final decision must rest with your physician.

Loss of consciousness (syncope)

Sudden loss of consciousness is a relatively frequent reason for a cardiology consultation. Some instances are trivial, but some may signal serious disorders. The following is a typical description of syncopal episode:

Doctor, I think that I fainted yesterday. I mean, I was walking from my bedroom to the kitchen and suddenly I found myself lying on the floor with a bruise on my forehead. After that I felt dizzy and weak but later on I recovered. I am perfectly well now, but I am frightened that it might happen again.

Although sometimes benign in nature, sudden loss of consciousness (syncope), especially if accompanied by a fall, is indeed a serious event which warrants medical attention. Reproducible occurrences clearly related to a precipitating factor, such as the following examples, may not warrant a full medical examination:

◆ blood-taking

◆ witnessing a stressful event

◆ sudden change in position from lying down to standing, especially if associated with dehydration and old age or use of a new medication to lower blood pressure.

On the other hand, unexplained syncope should prompt a detailed medical assessment, especially if associated with body injury or known cardiac disease. The patient should undergo a cardiac assessment, mainly to exclude either extremely low heart rate (bradycardia) or a severe rhythm disturbance.

Types of assessment

Continuous electrocardiographic (ECG) monitoring

The first screening study is generally continuous 24-hour ambulatory ECG monitoring (a Holter test). A detailed explanation of how ambulatory ECG recording is performed is given in Chapter 3.

However, since syncopal episodes may be sporadic, the Holter test may fail to identify the cause of the attacks, so a longer recording period (a few days) may be necessary.

Continuous loop recorder

In selected cases a more sophisticated method is to implant under the patient's skin a small recording device, called a continuous loop recorder (Figure 2.1), that will continuously record the heart rhythm for long periods of time (more than a year if necessary) and save arrhythmia episodes on its memory. The device can be interrogated after a new episode of fainting to see if any rhythm disturbance had been recorded.

Echocardiography

Organic cardiac pathology such as decreased ventricular function, cardiomyopathy, or severe valvular disease should be ruled out, so echocardiography is also frequently performed in these patients. A detailed explanation of echocardiography is given in Chapter 3.

If, by any of these means, a slow heart rate is found to be the cause of the syncope, a pacemaker will solve the problem. If severe rhythm disturbances are found, the patient may need an implantable defibrillator that will give an electric discharge to stabilize the cardiac rhythm when necessary. More information about each of these treatments can be found in Section 3 of this book.

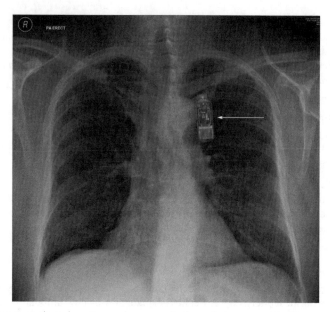

Figure 2.1 Implanted continuous loop recorder (arrow) as seen on chest X-ray.

Tilt tests

A relatively common form of syncope repeatedly occurs, without any apparent trigger, while standing. These patients may have normal hearts but an inappropriate blood pressure and/or heart response to prolonged standing. This is known as neurogenically mediated syncope and, when suspected because of the conditions of occurrence, it is further investigated with a tilt test. During a tilt test, the patient is strapped to a table which is then mechanically tilted to an almost vertical position for 20–40 minutes, while the blood pressure and an electrocardiogram are continuously recorded. A significant drop in blood pressure confirms the diagnosis.

Shortness of breath (dyspnoea)

Shortness of breath (SOB) is a frequently encountered symptom in heart disease, where it can be related to heart failure or some forms of angina. However, it is in no way specific to heart conditions, being associated with lung disease and obesity, among others. The diagnosis is further compounded by the frequent coexistence of these conditions in the same individual. A clear relationship to exercise, lack of a background of pulmonary disease, and the presence of some specific features, such as clear worsening when lying down and waking up at night because of sudden dyspnoea, support a cardiac origin. Frequently, however, the diagnosis cannot be made on clinical grounds alone.

Leg swelling (oedema)

Leg oedema is a frequent reason to refer a patient for cardiac evaluation because of suspected heart failure. Indeed, leg swelling is a common feature of advanced heart failure because of water retention and a rise in the venous pressure, resulting in passage of blood plasma out of the blood vessels. Typical cardiac oedema is bilateral and pitting in nature (a mark persist for a long time after applying local pressure). However, leg swelling is quite a common finding, which is also encountered in numerous non-cardiac conditions such as:

- obesity
- venous disease, especially after an acute venous inflammation of the deep veins (thrombophlebitis)
- nephrotic syndrome (loss of protein in urine, resulting in low protein levels in blood)
- lymphoedema due to poor lymphatic rather than venous drainage, resulting in hard oedema
- use of certain medications, such as amlodipine (see Chapter 13)
- idiopathic (unexplained), especially in women.

As an isolated finding, leg oedema is unlikely to be cardiac in nature, especially if it is asymmetrical and non-pitting, and a good response to diuretics does not necessarily confirm a cardiac cause.

3

Cardiac tests

The stethoscope and the heart sounds

Blood passes through the heart at velocities that normally range between 0.5 and 1.5 metres per second, sequentially opening and closing the four cardiac valves at a rate of 60–90 times per minute. The noise generated by so much mechanical activity can be heard, and listening to it can help a doctor to decide if the 'heart engine' is working normally or not.

Normal heart activity is heard as regular cycles of coupled sounds marking the closure and opening of the heart valves. Normal blood flowing through the heart is also sometimes heard as a faint murmur. Abnormal heart sounds or noisy murmurs will alert your doctor to the possibility of heart disease, with valvular heart diseases being the easiest to recognize in this way.

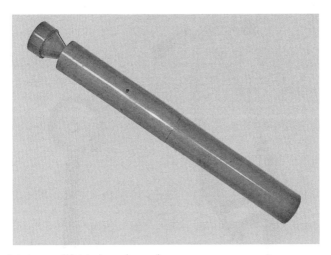

Figure 3.1 Laennec's original wooden stethoscope.
(Reproduced with kind permission of Medical Antiques Online http://www.antique.
med.com/)

Heart sounds are quite weak, so one has to literally put one's ear on the patient's chest in order to hear them. This is quite awkward and may be unacceptable, especially for female patients. This problem was solved by a nineteenth century French physician called Rene Laennec who showed that heart sounds can be amplified and distinctly heard by resting a wooden cylinder over the patient's chest (the Greek word for chest is *stethos)* and listening at the opposite end. This was the first stethoscope (Figure 3.1). The design of modern stethoscopes is much more sophisticated and ergonomic, but the principle remains the same (Figure 3.2).

The electrocardiogram and the electrical activity of the heart

As you know by now, the heart is actually a muscle. As with all body muscles, its mechanical activity is controlled by electrical currents that can be detected by specialized equipment. The graphical display of this electrical activity is the electrocardiogram (ECG), which is obtained using an electrocardiography machine. Pioneered in 1900 in the Netherlands by Einthowen, who was awarded the Nobel Prize for developing it, this technique is today the mainstay of any cardiological evaluation. The ECG is acquired by connecting the patient's arms and six well-defined locations on the chest to 10 cables (Figure 3.3) which conduct the electric currents of the heart to the ECG machine where, after filtering and amplification, the ECG tracing is obtained. The procedure is

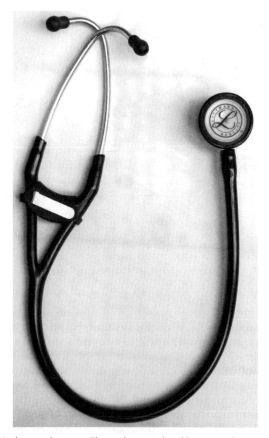

Figure 3.2 Modern stethoscope. The stethoscope head has a membrane on one side and a bell-like opening on the other side to allow selective amplification of high- and low-pitched sounds.

totally harmless and takes a few minutes to perform. The resulting ECG tracing will display some characteristic waves that mirror the electrical activity of the heart (Figure 3.4). The diagnostic value of the ECG is maximal for rhythm disturbances and for various forms of ischaemic heart disease, such as acute or old myocardial infarction. The ECG can also provide clues about other abnormalities, such as a thick cardiac muscle or predisposition to cardiac arrhythmias. However, this is not a foolproof tool. Remember:

◆ patients with diseased hearts can have innocent-looking ECGs

◆ absolutely normal individuals can exhibit apparently abnormal ECG tracings.

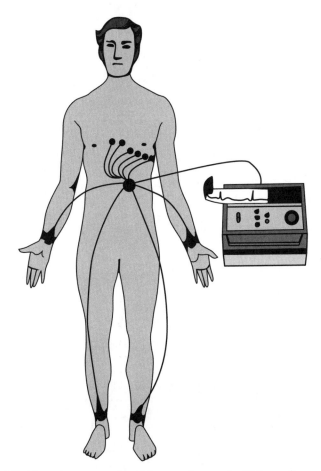

Figure 3.3 Schematic representation of the setup for a routine ECG recording: Electrodes are positioned on the four extremities and on ten defined positions on the chest and connected to the ECG machine.

Exercise test

A cardiologist is frequently confronted with the challenge of deciding whether a patient's complaints reflect underlying heart disease. The typical case is when the patient complains of chest pain, and the question is whether coronary disease is present but other exercise-related symptoms, such as weakness, shortness of breath, dizziness, or palpitations, may also warrant a cardiological work-up. The rationale of an exercise test is to subject the patient to a standardized effort and to note his/her symptoms, exercise capacity, blood pressure, pulse response, and electrocardiographic changes. The test is performed by

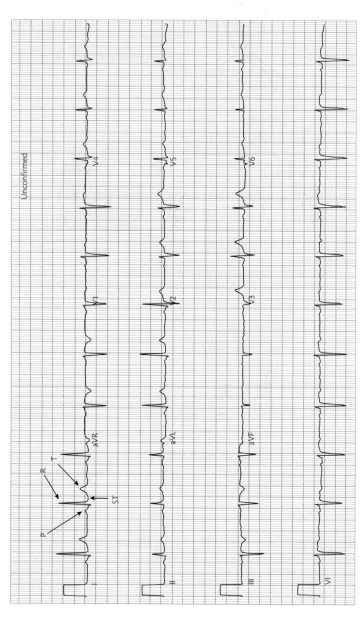

Figure 3.4 Normal ECG tracing. The small P waves reflect the atrial contraction and the tall R waves correspond to ventricular contraction. The T wave and the ST segment may change during, among others, myocardial ischaemia. Each P and R group of waves reflects a cardiac contraction.

having the patient exercise on a treadmill or stationary bicycle while he/she is connected to an ECG recorder and a blood pressure measurement apparatus. A standard protocol is used whereby the intensity of the effort is increased at fixed time intervals by changing the inclination and speed of the treadmill or the resistance to pedalling. For a test to be diagnostic in the assessment of coronary artery disease, a minimum age-derived heart rate should be achieved. A qualified technician performs the test, and a physician is not necessarily present in the test room although he/she should be readily available. Most places will provide you with a short leaflet instructing you on how to prepare for the test. As general guidance:

- Refrain from food intake and smoking for at least 3 hours before the test.
- Clarify with your doctor whether to take your medication as usual.
- If you have diabetes, ask for special guidance about timing of medication and food.
- Seek advice if you do not feel fit for the test on that particular day, because of flu or any other ailment.
- Wear comfortable loose clothing and light footwear, suitable for light running. Women should wear a bra.

The overall safety of the test is excellent, once some contraindications such as severe valvular disease or heart failure are excluded. Although exercise-induced symptoms and blood pressure response are also noted, the results of the test are based mainly on the ECG changes and are reported as:

- negative, i.e. normal (no findings)
- positive, i.e. abnormal
- non-conclusive, i.e. non-diagnostic.

You should be aware that, while this is an excellent and very low risk screening test, its overall accuracy is not very high and a negative result in a person with coronary artery disease (false-negative result) or of positive result in a healthy individual (false-positive result) is by no means rare. It is up to your doctor to decide whether to accept the test results as they are or to order a new one combined with either echocardiography or a nuclear study (see below).

Ambulatory ECG monitoring

A patient can occasionally experience worrisome symptoms of palpitations or irregular heartbeat and yet have no objective findings when seen in clinic. As already mentioned, some of these symptoms may be of no clinical significance, but occasionally they may reveal a serious disorder. An accurate diagnosis requires the objective visualization of the heart activity when they occur, which is difficult because of their very unpredictable and short-lived nature. In the 1950s Norman Holter, an American scientist, envisaged a method of solving this problem in which the patient wears a portable ECG recording device for a period of time, usually 24 hours, to allow for continuous ECG recording (Holter monitoring). The first machines were cumbersome, but modern devices are small, light, and unobtrusive to wear (Figure 3.5). The patient is encouraged to have a normal activity day and has to write down any cardiac symptoms and the time of their occurrence. Later on, this 'diary' is compared with the recorded ECG (Figure 3.6) to find out whether his/her symptoms reflect arrhythmia. Possible indications for this test include:

◆ palpitations

◆ dizzy spells

◆ unexplained syncope.

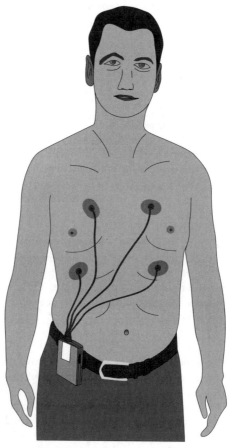

Figure 3.5 Holter monitoring. The device, cables, and electrodes are covered by clothes and allow normal activities.

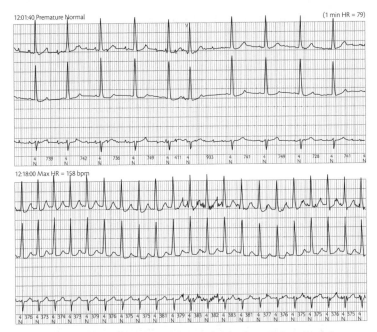

Figure 3.6 Diagnostic Holter recording: At 12:01 (upper three ECG tracings) the cardiac rhythm is normal. At 12:18 (lower three ECG tracings), at the time marked by the patient in his diary as 'strong palpitations', a rapid (160 beats/minute) heart rhythm is noted. In this case, Holter monitoring established the diagnosis of symptomatic paroxysmal supraventricular tachycardia.

If the symptoms are rare, and thus possibly missed in a random 24-hour monitoring period, a similar device can be used to extend the monitoring interval to 5–7 days. Alternatively, the technology exists for the patient to transmit his/her ECG at the time of the symptoms through a telephone to a diagnostic and monitoring centre.

The echocardiogram

Structural changes of the heart muscle and/or valves occur in many heart diseases (Table 3.1). These changes, and many others, can be demonstrated using echocardiography, which is a method to image the heart using ultrasound. Pioneered in the early 1950s by Inge Edler, a Swedish physician, echocardiography is today the most versatile, powerful, and readily available non-invasive diagnostic tool in cardiology. Impressive technological advances have expanded the diagnostic capabilities of this method to cover practically every cardiac pathology.

Table 3.1 Typical structural findings encountered in some common heart conditions

Disease	Structural change
Infarction	The affected heart wall area becomes thin and fibrotic and does not contract
Advanced heart failure	The heart is enlarged, the walls are thin, and the chambers are contracting poorly
Stenotic valve	The valve is thickened, with reduced mobility, and blood flows through it with increased velocity
Pericardial effusion	Fluid is seen around the heart

How does it work?

A focused ultrasound beam is directed to the heart and the reflected signal is used to display real-time two-dimensional (Figure 3.7) or, more recently, even three-dimensional images of the beating heart. The direction and velocity of the blood flowing through the heart cavities can also be imaged. The images are stored on tape or digitally for subsequent revision.

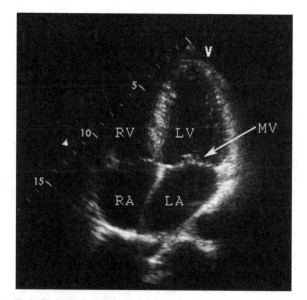

Figure 3.7 Typical echocardiographic image of a normal heart. Ventricular contractility and valve motion can easily be assessed when moving real-time images are displayed. LA, left atrium; LV, left ventricle; MV, mitral valve; RV, right ventricle.

How is it performed?

Most echo studies are performed by placing a small device that emits and receives ultrasound (transducer) over the patient's chest. The technique is known as transthoracic (from Latin *thorax*: chest) echocardiography (TTE). Expect to be asked to uncover your chest and lie on your left side. The technician or physician performing the study will connect you to ECG cables and, after applying some gel to a small transducer, will position it on your chest at various locations to obtain the echocardiographic images. The whole study should not take more than 10–15 minutes and you should experience no discomfort except for occasional light chest pressure from the transducer and the 'cold' feeling of the gel.

Is there any risk involved?

Absolutely none. Based on huge experience accumulated worldwide, there is no evidence of damage related to echocardiographic examinations. Remember that the same technology is safely used in pregnant women to visualize the foetus whose tissues are much more sensitive than those of an adult person.

Special echocardiographic techniques

Transoesophageal echocardiography (TOE)

If it is necessary to obtain higher-quality images of the heart or to visualize cardiac or vascular structures which are suboptimally imaged with TTE, it is possible to place a specially designed transducer into the patient's oesophagus (gullet). Having the transducer situated in the immediate proximity of the heart without the interposition of the chest wall allows images of superb quality to be obtained. A spray provides local anaesthesia in the oral cavity and the throat, and mild intravenous sedation is frequently used, so that, overall, the study should not involve more than slight discomfort in experienced hands. Also, the risks involved are minimal. TOE is not a routine examination but it is widely used for special cases such as:

- cardiological examination after a stroke
- suspected infection of the valves (endocarditis)
- suspected malfunction of prosthetic valves
- assessment before cardiac valve surgery
- suspected disease of the aorta.

If you are referred for a TOE you will receive detailed instructions on how to prepare for it. For your general information, you should:

- fast for 4–6 hours
- inform your physician or the team performing the TOE about:
  - allergies

◆ diseases of the digestive system, especially ulcer, digestive system bleeding, or trouble in swallowing

◆ arrange for someone to accompany you since you may feel slightly dizzy afterwards and, if given sedation, you will not be allowed to drive.

Stress echocardiography

You know by now that the regular exercise test performed to detect coronary artery disease can be unreliable in some cases. A simple way to improve its accuracy is to look not only at ECG changes but also at the echocardiogram before and after exercise. A decrease in the contractility of the heart after exercise is indicative of disease. The test relies on side-by-side comparison of images before and after stress, but for the patient it is a simple exercise test with an echocardiographic examination performed before and immediately after exercise. For individuals who are not able to exercise, so-called pharmacological tests are available where a drug is administered that will mimic the cardiac effects of physical exertion (Figure 3.8). The most widely used drug for stress echocardiography is dobutamine. The test is very safe and generally well tolerated, although you may experience headache, palpitations, and some general discomfort during the infusion.

Nuclear studies

Although there are many technical variants, basically there are two kinds of nuclear studies relevant to the cardiac patient.

Myocardial perfusion studies

In this technique, which is frequently known as a 'thallium exercise test' or MIBI scan, the patient performs a regular exercise and, at peak exercise, a radioactive thallium isotope is injected into a peripheral vein. The thallium isotope enters the cardiac cells, and imaging the heart with a gamma camera will provide a mapped image of the cardiac muscle blood perfusion during exercise. The heart is imaged at rest and then after exercise for comparison. Local routines vary: some laboratories may complete the whole study in one day (allow for 4–6 hours), and others may perform it in two stages on two consecutive days. This a much more accurate (although not totally fail-safe) method of assessing coronary blood supply than using the ECG during a regular exercise test. However, it is also much more expensive and time consuming, so it is reserved for those cases where the regular exercise test is inconclusive. The test may also be used for persons who are unable to exercise; in this case, the imaging is combined with administration of a drug that will obviate the need for physical exertion (usually dipyridamole). As for a regular exercise test, the only thing necessary to get ready for this test is to avoid food intake for a few hours (some places require fasting after midnight if the test is scheduled for early morning) and to check with your physician which, if any, of your regular medicines you

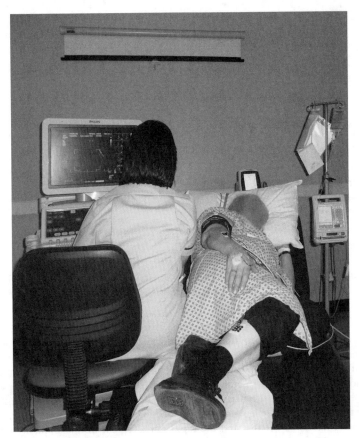

Figure 3.8 Standard set-up for pharmacological stress echo. The drug is delivered by an infusion pump, while the patient's ECG and blood pressure are continuously monitored and echo images are acquired.

are allowed to take. For dipyridamole studies you should not drink coffee or tea for 24 hours before the test and you should inform your physician if you suffer from asthma or bronchitis.

Nuclear ventriculography

Ventricular function assessment by echocardiography is reliable and should be used in most cases. If the need arises in selected cases, nuclear ventriculography (MUGA) can be used to quantify the contraction strength of your heart more accurately by injecting a radioactive tracer (technetium) and imaging the heart with a gamma camera. The results are given as an ejection fraction (EF), i.e. how much of the blood filling the heart is ejected into the aorta during systole. In a healthy individual the ejection fraction should be above 55%.

 Frequently Asked Question

Q: My GP received the results of my recent MIBI scan and told me that it was negative so I had no reason to worry. I am confused now. I thought that 'negative' was something bad.

A: In medical jargon, 'negative' means 'no findings' and 'positive' means findings are present'. So, generally, a negative test is a good or normal one, while a positive one may be a reason for concern. If in doubt, you can ask your doctor to clarify this.

Advanced imaging techniques

Modern computed tomography (CT) and magnetic resonance imaging (MRI) are highly sophisticated imaging modalities used in many medical fields, including cardiology.

CT uses X-rays and advanced computer processing to generate high-quality 'sliced' images, but lacks 'functional' information (heart contractility, valve disease) and therefore, except for selected cases of aortic pathology, is not a routine tool for cardiac investigation. A sophisticated development of CT technology (CT angiography) allows accurate evaluation of the coronary arteries. Its exact role in the assessment of patients with coronary artery disease is under continuous revision, reflecting rapidly occurring technical advances. The non-invasive nature of the test and the rapid improvement in image quality may support CT angiography as a lower-risk alternative to standard invasive angiography. However, the amount of iodine-based contrast is similar to that needed during standard angiography and the radiation exposure may be even higher, although recent technological advances make this less of a concern. As things stand now, CT angiography may be considered instead of standard angiography in patients with intermediate risk of coronary disease and in selected cases after coronary bypass graft surgery.

Cardiac MRI uses exposure to intense magnetic fields and changes in the electromagnetic field of the body tissues to produce superb-quality images of heart and blood vessels. Image quality and resolution are superior to echocardiography, and, unlike CT, functional information is provided as well. However, the routine use of cardiac MRI is limited by high costs, lack of availability as a 'bedside' procedure, and limitations on its use in the presence of mechanical implants, especially pacemakers. Cardiac MR is used when alternative imaging methods cannot provide accurate information with a high degree of confidence.

Cardiac catheterization

This is a method in which the coronary arteries are directly visualized (angiography), so the question of whether they are diseased or not can be answered with an almost total degree of certitude. Catheterization also allows direct measurement of intra-cardiac pressures and gradients, which is useful for valvular diseases, although in these cases echocardiography is now considered the main diagnostic method. Therefore, when speaking about catheterization, what is generally meant is angiography.

When is catheterization used?

The answer is not a rigid one (although guidelines do exist), and the decision whether to perform angiography in a particular case will reflect both established practice and the individual approach of your cardiologist. The following is a list of situations for which angiography may be considered:

◆ symptoms suspected to be cardiac in origin when non-invasive tests fail to give a clear answer

◆ suspected or known coronary disease when the patient is considered to be at high risk according to the clinical picture or the results of non-invasive tests

◆ a change for the worse in the clinical picture of a patient with known coronary disease

◆ selected cases of acute myocardial infarction or similarly unstable and potentially dangerous conditions.

How to prepare for the catheterization. Am I going to spend the night in the hospital?

You will probably receive detailed instructions from the medical team taking care of you. In the unlikely case that you do not:

◆ Let them know about any medical allergy you may have, especially to anaesthetics, iodine, fish, or seafood.

◆ Find out whether you should take your medicines as usual before entering the hospital.

◆ As a rule, the procedure is performed after a 6-hours fasting period.

◆ You may be instructed to shave your groin area.

◆ Expect to receive light sedation before being taken to the catheterization suite.

Whether or not you have to spend a night in hospital following the procedure is highly variable. Simple cases may be admitted on the day of the scheduled procedure, while other patients, such as those with renal failure or receiving anticoagulant therapy, may be asked to enter the hospital earlier. After the catheterization, expect to be discharged the next day, although same-day discharge is occasionally practised in uncomplicated cases.

How is this done? What to expect

You will lie on the catheterization table, connected to an ECG monitor and covered with sterile drapes except for the area used to enter a peripheral artery, usually either the femoral artery (in the groin) or the radial artery (in the wrist), which will be cleaned and scrubbed and left uncovered. The operator will give you a local anaesthetic shot and then will locate the artery by palpation. This artery will be punctured with a hollow needle through which a special wire will be passed. The wire will guide a catheter, i.e. a specially designed hollow tube, into the artery. The whole procedure should be painless. Once in the artery, the catheter is advanced under fluoroscopic (X-ray) guidance to the openings of the coronary arteries (Figure 3.9) and contrast material is injected so that the

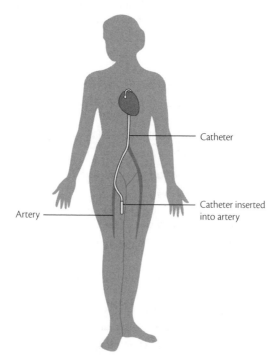

Figure 3.9 Schematic representation of cardiac catheterization. In this case, the catheter is introduced through the right femoral artery and advanced to the opening of a coronary artery.

(Reproduced with the kind permission of the British Heart Foundation, the copyright owner)

arteries can be visualized and images recorded for later inspection. You are fully conscious during the procedure and you can communicate with the team and even see the images of your arteries on the monitor.

What happens afterwards?

If the angiogram shows normal vessels, the procedure ends at this stage and a plug made of slowly absorbable biological material is placed at the site of the puncture, allowing early mobilization, discharge, and resumption of normal activities within a few days. Alternatively, local pressure is applied, either manually or using a sandbag or special device, for 20–30 minutes. If the angiogram does show diseased vessels (Figure 3.10), the operator will discuss with you the available options, i.e. whether continuing medical treatment is an option or whether the vessels should be opened using balloons and stents or surgically bypassed. Depending on the particular case and local routines, the balloon procedure may be performed immediately or you may be brought back for it at a later date.

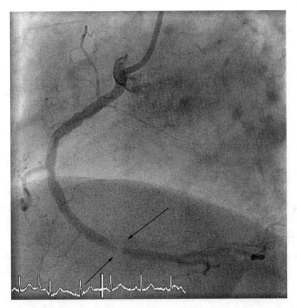

Figure 3.10 Tight stenosis (arrows) in the right coronary artery, demonstrated by angiography.

Cardiac Tests: Frequently Asked Questions

Test results

Q: After I completed my test I asked the technician whether the results were good but he refused to comment and would only say that the results would be forwarded to my doctor and he would answer all my questions. I am due to see my doctor in three weeks and I am concerned. I am afraid that the results were not good and the technician did not want to worry me.

A: You should not worry, the technician did exactly what he was supposed to do, irrespective of the results. Some tests need later review, results may be borderline, others require a good integration of all data to be correctly interpreted, so the accepted policy is not to offer an opinion. Though some technicians may occasionally convey a general reassuring message about the results of the study, they are not supposed to discuss them. Don't assume anything if you are not given an immediate answer to your questions, wait to see your doctor. Just rest reassured that if anything requiring an urgent evaluation is found out during the study, the technician will take the necessary steps.

Tests safety

Q: My cardiologist referred me to an exercise MIBI scan. At first I was glad that perhaps I wouldn't need an angiogram, but then I began to worry: Is it safe to inject a radioactive substance?

A: You should not worry. Some tests, such as CTs, angiograms, or nuclear studies, involve a higher exposure level than a regular chest X-ray examination, but the absolute amount is still small and there is no evidence of long-term damage. It is accepted that the clear benefit of a detailed diagnosis far outweighs any potential and unproved risk. If you have a history of previous multiple tests involving radiation exposure, you should inform your physician. Special considerations are needed in children, pregnant, or breastfeeding women.

After the tests

Q: I complained of swollen legs to my GP who referred me for an echocardiographic scan. I understand that the report will be sent back to him. What happens next? I fully trust my GP, but maybe only a specialist can understand the results?

A: The report will definitely be sent to your GP, not only as courtesy but mainly because he knows you and has a broad perspective of your case. Although, as you suspect, the report may contain many 'technicalities', it also always includes a summary providing clinical information. It will be your GP's decision whether to seek advice from a cardiologist. Also, local routines may vary, but if a significant finding is uncovered by the test, the report is likely to include a recommendation that a cardiological consultation is advised.

4

Risk factors that increase the possibility of heart disease

 Key Points

- There are a variety of factors and conditions that can affect your chances of suffering from heart disease.
- Age, gender, and heredity are non-changeable risk factors.
- Smoking, hypertension, and hypercholesterolaemia are modifiable risk factors.

A variety of conditions have been associated with cardiovascular diseases, and therefore they are defined as risk factors. For some, the causal mechanism is quite clear; for others, it is more of an observational association. The main cardiovascular risk factors are listed below and are discussed further in this chapter.

- Major non-changeable risk factors:
  - age
  - gender
  - heredity.
- Major changeable risk factors:
  - smoking
  - high blood cholesterol levels (hypercholesterolaemia)
  - high blood pressure (arterial hypertension)
  - physical inactivity
  - overweight
  - diabetes mellitus.
- Contributing risk factors:
  - psychological stress.

Age and gender, family history, and race

Advanced age is associated with increased frequency of cardiovascular diseases. More than 80% of people who die of coronary disease are older than 65 years. Also, the average age for a first heart attack is in the 'elderly range', which is around 65 years in men and 70 years in women, although the age can be much lower if risk factors are also present.

Female gender is considered to have a cardiovascular protective effect, and clinical coronary disease is rare in pre-menopausal women, possibly because of a protective effect of feminine hormones. There is a definite increase in cardiovascular mortality in post-menopausal women, although it remains below that encountered in men until the late seventies.

Finally, both family history and race correlate with cardiovascular risk. A positive family history is defined as the presence of coronary disease in first-degree relatives (mother, father, sibling, offspring) below the age of 55 years for males and 65 years for females.

Individuals of African or South Asian descent have higher rates of cardiovascular disease than Caucasians. Although people from the same family or the same sociocultural background may share same changeable risk factors, the relation described above persists even after taking these into account.

Age, gender, and heredity are obviously non-modifiable risk factors. Their importance resides in 'flagging' individuals at high risk, thus justifying higher awareness and the need for risk-factor modification in cases that otherwise would be considered borderline.

❓ Frequently Asked Question

Q: I am 70 years old and I have just had a heart attack. My children are in their thirtiess. Does it mean that there is heart disease in the family? Should they be concerned and have some tests?

A: No, heart attacks at your age are not unusual, so they are not considered to represent a familial trait. As recommended to all adults, your children should maintain a healthy lifestyle and have a risk-factor profile assessment, but otherwise there is no need to be worried.

Smoking

Over 4000 chemical compounds are present in tobacco smoke. The main ones, relevant for their possible health damaging effects, are as follows.

- Nicotine: an alkaloid that may increase heart rate and blood pressure and is responsible for developing smoking 'addiction'.

◆ Tar: compounds resulting from burning tobacco. Tar has toxic effects on the lungs and mucosa of the oral cavity.

◆ Carbon monoxide: a gas that competes with oxygen for blood transport.

Cigarette smoking has a strong association with chronic bronchitis, lung cancer, and cardiovascular diseases. Half of all long-term smokers will eventually die of a smoking-related disease. Cardiac mortality is two to three times higher in smokers compared with non-smokers, and the odds for graft closure after bypass surgery are also higher in smokers. Possible mechanisms include:

◆ increased tendency for vascular spasm (contraction of the arteries)

◆ lower levels of 'good' cholesterol

◆ greater adhesiveness of blood platelets and thus increased tendency for blood clotting.

There is no 'safe' smoking level, but risk is higher in heavy smokers (more than 20 cigarettes/day), in individuals below 50 years of age, and in association with other risk factors or special conditions such as diabetes or women using oral contraceptives. Cigarette smoking is a leading preventable cause of cardiovascular disease, and smoking cessation significantly lowers cardiovascular risk.

Smoking cessation is a major target for reducing cardiovascular and lung diseases rates. The motivation to quit smoking is a prerequisite, but quitters can be helped by:

◆ being educated about the effects of smoking

◆ attending support groups

◆ nicotine replacement therapy (NRT), i.e. nicotine delivered by chewing gum or transdermal patches so that nicotine withdrawal symptoms are manageable without the damage of tar and carbon monoxide related to actual smoking

◆ Specific drugs such as buprion: an antidepressant which helps the individual to cope with nicotine withdrawal.

 Frequently Asked Question

Q: After 20 years of smoking about 20 cigarettes a day, I managed to give up and in fact it is easier than I expected. Is my risk of heart disease going down now or it will remain always higher than that of a lifetime non-smoker?

A: Yes, your coronary artery disease and stroke risk are steadily decreasing, although it can take 10–15 years before it is the same as those of a similar age- and gender-matched lifetime non-smoker. Also, the younger the age at which you give up smoking, the higher the benefit.

High cholesterol levels

People with high levels of blood fats (lipids) are at increased risk of coronary artery disease. The classification of blood lipids is quite complex, but for practical purposes the two kinds of fats that we are talking about are cholesterol and triglycerides.

The strongest association with coronary disease has been proved for cholesterol, which is therefore defined as a major modifiable risk factor and a target for intervention. Cholesterol is a lipid whose name reflects its structure, i.e. carbon atoms linked in rings (sterols) (Figure 4.1). Cholesterol is present in food but the main source of body cholesterol is its liver synthesis from saturated (animal and dairy) fats present in our diet.

Although this chapter focuses on the negative impact of high cholesterol levels on cardiovascular health, cholesterol is an important component of cell walls and is essential for the synthesis of steroid hormones. In order to be transported in blood, cholesterol is incorporated in complex molecules called lipoproteins. There are five types of lipoproteins, and cholesterol is incorporated mainly in two of them which differ in density and molecular weight: low-density lipoproteins (LDLs) and high-density lipoproteins (HDLs).

Elevated cholesterol is considered a strong risk factor for coronary artery disease, but in fact only the LDL-cholesterol (bad cholesterol) is associated with certain types of heart disease and HDL-cholesterol may actually have a protective effect (good cholesterol). Therefore the value of the LDL-cholesterol and the ratio of total cholesterol to HDL-cholesterol are taken into account along with the total cholesterol level when cardiovascular risk is assessed.

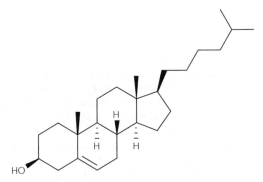

Figure 4.1 Chemical structure of cholesterol.

What are the normal cholesterol values and what is high cholesterol?

The average cholesterol level in adult individuals is about 5 mmol/litre (190 mg%) and an ideal level would be less than that. However, as discussed in chapter 3 the decision to initiate specific treatment to lower cholesterol levels takes into account the overall risk factors burden and the full lipid profile rather than the absolute cholesterol level.

Why do some people have high cholesterol levels (hypercholesterolaemia)?

In secondary hypercholesterolaemia, cholesterol levels are elevated due to other clearly identifiable diseases or conditions, such as hypothyroidism (insufficient production of thyroid hormone by the thyroid gland), some forms of renal disease, or excessive alcohol consumption.

In primary hypercholesterolaemia, cholesterol levels are elevated even in the absence of these factors, representing a genetic predisposition. This form of hypercholesterolaemia is by far the most common. In extreme cases, a familial clustering of high cholesterol or coronary disease at a young age is encountered together with very high (>7.5 mmol/litre) cholesterol levels. This is known as familial hypercholesterolaemia and is thought to affect about 1 in 500 of the European population. For further information, contact Heart UK.

Triglycerides are chemical compounds including three fatty acids linked to a molecule of glycerol. They represent the main chemical form of lipid storage and their blood concentration raises rapidly after a fat-rich meal. Normal levels are ≤2 mmol/litre (177 mg%) after a 12-hour fasting period. Elevated triglycerides are frequently associated with other risk conditions, such as diabetes and obesity, but are less of a risk factor for coronary artery disease unless their level is very high. Also, lowering triglycerides with diet and exercise is easier than lowering cholesterol.

Management of hypercholesterolaemia

There is strong evidence that lowering cholesterol will prevent a cardiac event in those without apparent heart disease (primary prevention) or a repeat event in those who already have manifest coronary disease (secondary prevention). Several drugs are currently available to lower blood lipids when diet is not enough. Statins are effective in lowering cholesterol and have been shown to decrease the risk of coronary artery disease, and fibrates are mainly used to lower triglycerides. These drugs are generally very well tolerated, but in high doses or in susceptible individuals they can induce muscle damage (see Chapter 13). The major cardiological organizations have published guidelines for desired lipid blood levels and the need for diet or drug therapy (see Appendix A).

Arterial hypertension (raised blood pressure)

Arterial hypertension is a common condition, with reported prevalences ranging from 30% to 60% in the 35–64 years age range in the Western world. Men are more commonly affected than women, and some ethnic groups such as Black Americans and African Caribbeans are particularly susceptible. The reported figures may in fact be an underestimation since many cases are not diagnosed. The frequency of hypertension rises exponentially with age and it is probably present in three-quarters of individuals above the age of 70.

Although, hypertension is occasionally secondary i.e. related to other identifiable and treatable conditions (usually specific forms of renal disease and some endocrine disorders), the vast majority of cases (> 90%) have no identifiable cause (primary hypertension) and are due to a yet to be defined combination of genetic predisposition and environmental factors. Hypertension is frequently found in association with other risk factors, such as obesity and diabetes.

How is blood pressure measured?

Blood pressure (BP) is measured in millimetres of mercury (mmHg) and is defined using two values: a higher one called systolic (i.e. the value of blood pressure at the time of the contraction of the left ventricle) and a lower one called diastolic (i.e. the value of the blood pressure at the time of ventricular relaxation). It is written down as a pair of numbers, e.g. 120/80 mmHg. Hypertension is diagnosed when any of these values is above the normal limit.

To measure blood pressure, a cuff is placed over the arm and the pressure in it is gradually increased until the flow in the brachial artery stops due to compression. Upon gradual release of the cuff pressure, the blood flow through the artery resumes when the cuff pressure equals the highest blood pressure (systolic pressure) and becomes totally silent when the cuff pressure is lower than the lowest pressure (diastolic pressure). The resumption of flow is detected with a stethoscope placed over the brachial artery. By noting the cuff pressure at the appearance and the disappearance of blood flow sounds, the systolic and diastolic blood pressures are detected. Electronic devices use microphones or sensors incorporated into the cuff to detect the systolic and diastolic pressures.

Precautions to take when measuring the blood pressure

◆ BP is extremely responsive to psychological stress or physical activity. Therefore it should be measured with the patient in a comfortable sitting position, after at least 5 minutes of rest. At least two measurements should be taken a few minutes apart. In patients with elevated blood pressure in the mild range and an overall low cardiovascular risk, it is reasonable to repeat the blood pressure readings over a period of a few months before making a final diagnosis of hypertension.

- In individuals with large arms, cuffs of an appropriate size should be used to avoid spuriously high readings.

- BP measurements can be inaccurate in patients with irregular heart rates.

Hypertension: complications and management

Hypertension is a major contributor to cardiovascular disease, the risk of which increases continuously with raising BP, starting in the normal values range. The harmful effects of hypertension are related to its mechanical effects on the arterial wall, which aggravate and enhance the effects of other risk factors, such as smoking, diabetes, and hypercholesterolaemia, resulting in atherosclerosis (see Chapter 5).

Hypertension has also a damaging effect on the cardiac muscle, which becomes thicker and in the end may fail due to prolonged exposure to high levels of blood pressure.

When assessing the impact of hypertension, or deciding on treatment in borderline cases, the concept of 'target-organ damage' is used, i.e. evidence of injury in organs that are specifically affected by high BP levels. Looking for this evidence is part of the complete work-up of a hypertensive patient.

Target organs and specific damage due to hypertension

- Heart
  - coronary artery disease (angina, heart attack)
  - thickening of ventricular walls (hypertrophy) detected by ECG or echocardiography
  - left ventricular damage (may manifest as heart failure or be detected by echocardiography)
- Brain
  - stroke
  - dementia
- Peripheral vascular disease
  - arterial obstruction (generally: narrowing in legs arteries)
  - aortic aneurysms (dilatation of the aorta)
- Eyes
  - hypertensive retinopathy (changes in the blood vessels of the retina)
- Kidneys
  - chronic renal failure

What are the normal BP values and what is high blood pressure?

The definition of normal values (i.e. above which hypertension is diagnosed and treatment is considered) is somewhat arbitrary and dynamic, reflecting

Table 4.1 Cut-off limits for blood pressure values and hypertensive stages

	Systolic BP (mmHg)	Diastolic BP (mmHg)	Treatment needed
Normal BP	≤120	≤80	No
High normal/pre-hypertension	120–139	80–89	Possibly
Mild hypertension	140–159	90–99	Possibly
Moderate hypertension	160–179	100–109	Yes
Severe hypertension	≥180	≥110	Yes

our evolving knowledge about the impact of hypertension on cardiovascular health and the benefit of active treatment. Also, slight differences exist between recommendations of various medical bodies (Table 4.1).

The high-normal or pre-hypertension range refers to BP readings that are still normal but warrant follow-up in selected cases, or, if the overall cardiovascular risk is high, may justify treatment.

White coat hypertension

Some individuals have consistently high BP readings in their doctor's office but normal values when BP is taken in different circumstances. If this condition, which has to do with the psychological stress of measuring BP in a formal medical environment, is suspected and there is no evidence of target-organ damage, the patient can be further assessed using a device for automated 24-hour ambulatory BP monitoring or can be encouraged to measure his/her own BP using one of the commercially available BP measuring devices. Of note, the accepted levels for diagnosing hypertension by automated or self-measurement are slightly lower than those obtained by standard measurements.

Treatment of hypertension

Good control of BP may lower the risk of stroke by up to 40% and the risk of coronary disease by up to 25%. The decision to use specific anti-hypertensive drugs (see Chapter 12) is based on actual BP measurements, total risk factors profile, and coexistent diseases. Irrespective of the medication used, a few principles are valid in most patients.

- Lifestyle modification is an integral part of hypertension management and in mild cases can be sufficient to achieve BP control. The main targets of lifestyle modification for BP control are the following.
  - Reduced salt intake: a simple practical approach is not to add salt when cooking or at table and to avoid processed food and salted snacks.
  - Weight loss.
  - Exercise: you can start with just brisk walking a few times a week.
- Any associated risk factors should be treated as appropriate.

- If specific medication is used for lowering BP:
  - Most available anti-hypertensive drugs are of similar potency. The decision to use one rather than the other relates to the existence of associated diseases or expected benefits or limitations in your particular case:
    - ACE inhibitors are practically 'a must' if diabetes or heart failure are also present
    - beta-blockers are a good option if angina or arrhythmias are also present, but are less efficient as anti-hypertensives in the elderly or in patients of African descent and are contraindicated in asthmatic patients
    - diuretics and calcium-channel blockers are a good option in uncomplicated cases, especially in the elderly.
  - While mild cases can be controlled with one drug only, the majority of anti-hypertensive patients will need two or three medications. This is not a major inconvenience since most available drugs can be taken once a day. 'Combo' pills can also be used when appropriate.
  - Severe resistant cases may require specialist input to manage more aggressive treatments and to rule out the rare cases of secondary hypertension.

 Frequently Asked Questions

Q: I have been started on a tablet for high blood pressure and, though the readings are better now, it is still high on occasions. My doctor wants to add a second medication. I really hate taking pills, so couldn't I just have a higher dose of what I am already taking?

A: Available data show that most patients will need more than just one drug to achieve good blood pressure control. The general approach is that it is better to use two drugs at smaller doses to avoid the side effects related to high doses. Obviously, the decision has to be flexible and adapted to each particular case, so you can discuss this with your doctor. Also, combinations of drugs in one tablet are available and this can keep the number of pills you are taking low.

Q: I was started on anti-hypertensive drugs a year ago and now my blood pressure is perfectly normal and I feel well and fit. I have no other health problems. Can I stop my medication?

A: Most likely, no. Your blood pressure is normal now because of the drugs. If your hypertension was mild only and since then you lost weight and exercise regularly, you could give it a try, but the odds of recurrence are high. In any case, consult your GP.

Physical inactivity (sedentarism)

Physical inactivity is associated not only with cardiovascular diseases but also with other conditions such as diabetes, obesity, osteoporosis, and depression. Regular physical activity is credited with decreasing cardiovascular mortality by up to 35%. The mechanisms involved are complex but physical activity improves vascular wall function and helps to normalize blood pressure, lipid profile, and blood sugar levels. In fact, mild cases of diabetes, hypertension, or hyperlipidaemia can be managed through lifestyle changes including physical activity.

According to recent guidelines, healthy adults should engage in 30 minutes of moderate aerobic physical activity (brisk walking inducing an increase in heart rate) on at least 5days a week or 20 minutes of intense activity (jogging) on 3 days week (Table 4.2). Routine cardiovascular assessment and screening are not necessary in asymptomatic individuals with a low risk-factor profile before they engage in a programme of moderate activity. Elderly patients and those with known cardiovascular disease or any functional limitation should be assessed before starting a regular programme.

Obesity

Obesity is more than an aesthetic concern, although its social consequences and the impact on the self-image of affected individuals are not negligible. Obesity is due to a combination of a genetic predisposition and an unhealthy lifestyle, mainly sedentarism and a high-calorie high-fat diet rich in refined carbohydrates. For the last 30 years, the Western world has been faced with a real epidemic of obesity. An increase in prevalence from 12% to 18% was reported between 1991 and 1998 in the USA, and the reported present prevalence of obesity in the UK is 24%, a 15% increase from 1993 levels. Obesity is ubiquitous, but is more prevalent in the lower socioeconomic strata where not only is adherence to a healthy diet less likely but the social pressure of not being overweight may be less.

Table 4.2 Hourly metabolic equivalent of various daily and sport-related activities

Moderate physical activity (3–6 Mets)	Vigorous physical activity (>6 Mets)
Regular walking: 3 Mets	Jogging: 8–10 Mets
Brisk walking: 5 Mets	Running: 11 Mets
Light cycling on flat: 6 Mets	Moderate–fast cycling on flat: 8–10 Mets
Leisure swimming: 6 Mets	Moderate–hard swimming: 8–11 Mets
Golf: 4 Mets	

Met: metabolic unit (the energy needed for normal body functioning at rest).

Table 4.3 Diseases and conditions associated with obesity

Coronary artery disease
Arterial hypertension
Type 2 diabetes
Sleep apnoea
Venous insufficiency (resulting in leg oedema)
Venous thrombosis and pulmonary embolism
Depression
Certain cancers: breast, bowel, womb

Excess accumulation of adipose (fatty) tissue is associated with complex metabolic disorders, other cardiovascular risk factors, and an increased risk of coronary disease and also non-cardiovascular diseases (Table 4.3).

When is obesity diagnosed?

Obesity is diagnosed when actual weight is above that expected for the individual's height. The ratio of weight (in kilograms) to squared height (in metres) is known as body mass index (BMI) and defines the weight status of an individual (Table 4.4).

A special pattern of obesity, 'central obesity', relates to preferential fat storage around the abdomen rather than the hips or thighs. Central obesity is diagnosed at a waist circumference of more than 37 inches (94 cm) in men and more than 32 inches (80 cm) in women. Central obesity increases the cardiovascular risk more than the level derived from the BMI only. Therefore it is an important parameter of weight status assessment.

Obesity and cardiovascular risk

The relationship between obesity and cardiovascular disease is complex. It includes associated metabolic disorders, an increased inflammatory state, and

Table 4.4 Cut-off BMI values for normal weight and obesity grades

Weight status	BMI
Underweight	<18.5
Normal	18.5–24.9
Overweight	25–29.9
Obesity	≥30
I (mild)	30–35
II (moderate)	35–40
III (severe)	≥40

abnormal artery wall reactivity. In severe cases, direct harmful cardiac effects are noted, such as increased cardiac workload, heart chamber dilation, and fatty infiltration, possibly leading to heart failure. Obese patients are more likely to have concomitant cardiac risk factors, such as hypertension, diabetes, and dyslipidaemia, and their impact is increased by the overweight status. Also, from a practical point of view, physical examination may be limited, and symptoms such as fatigue, dyspnoea, and leg oedema are less specific and therefore more difficult to assess in obese individuals. As a result of its own direct effects and frequent association with other risk factors, obesity is strongly connected with an increased risk of stroke, early coronary disease, arrhythmias, and both cardiovascular and all-cause mortality.

Metabolic syndrome

The interrelationship between obesity and related conditions and their additive impact on the overall cardiovascular risk is illustrated by the concept of 'metabolic syndrome'. Metabolic syndrome is diagnosed when an individual presents with a combination of abnormalities as detailed below:

♦ central obesity

AND

♦ two of the following:
  ♦ high BP (≥130/85 mmHg) or present treatment for hypertension
  ♦ high triglyceride levels (1.7 mmol/litre) or present treatment
  ♦ low HDL-cholesterol levels (≤1 mmol/litre)
  ♦ high fasting blood glucose (≥ 5.6 mmol/litre) or diagnosed diabetes.

Losing weight

If you are overweight, as defined above, you should make weight loss a major health goal. Although a proper diet is central to any weight-loss programme, it is essential that it integrates with a full lifestyle change approach if possible. The following is a list of key points to remember if you are serious about losing weight. These suggestions focus on losing weight and not on specific diets for conditions such as diabetes or dyslipidaemia.

♦ Be 'calorie aware', i.e. have an idea of what your daily caloric intake is. Use food product description labels and available tables. For a steady weight loss, aim at no more than 1500–1800 cal/day, although individual variations are wide and depend on gender, body size, and activity level, so this figure is orientative only.

♦ Build your caloric intake on fruit, vegetables, and starchy foods (rice, pasta, bread (preferably whole grain)) for carbohydrates and on lean meat, fish, eggs, and beans for proteins. Avoid high-fat/high-sugar food and highly saturated fat products (butter, fat-rich cheese).

- Change your eating habits and develop an 'eating discipline'.
  - Eat regularly, have three meals daily including breakfast and avoid snacking.
  - Eat slowly.
  - Avoid overeating:
    - stop when you feel full
    - develop a culture of not eating an extra portion.
  - Be aware of apparently 'innocent' but nevertheless high-calorie foods: avocado, alcoholic beverages.
  - You may occasionally indulge yourself: eating out and family occasions.

Diabetes

Diabetes mellitus (DM) is a complex metabolic disorder, having at its core poor glucose (sugar) control. Blood glucose levels are controlled by insulin, a hormone produced by the pancreas.

Type 1 diabetes is an absolute lack of available insulin due to scarce synthesis, and onset is usually during childhood or young age. Type 1 diabetes is quite rare and is usually recognized by the rapid onset of highly suggestive symptoms such as thirst, passing increased amounts of urine (polyuria), and weight loss. In rare cases, the first manifestation is a severe potentially life-threatening complication—diabetic coma.

Type 2 diabetes is generally associated with middle-age onset and overweight, and is much more frequent (about 90% of all cases). However, when poorly controlled, it may present with symptoms similar to those of type 1 diabetes. It is generally asymptomatic and it is more likely to be discovered incidentally by blood tests performed as screening or when complications occur.

It is important to emphasize active screening in individuals at risk, especially patients over the age of 40, since type 2 diabetes may be present long before the symptoms appear. If you have reason to believe that you may be suffering from diabetes, the first step is to visit your GP for a consultation and a quick and easy blood test.

Diabetes and cardiovascular disease

Both type 1 and type 2 diabetes are associated with a significantly increased risk of cardiovascular complications (heart attack, heart failure, stroke, peripheral artery obstruction) which in diabetic patients occur earlier, develop more quickly, and are associated with higher mortality than in non-diabetic patients. The overall risk of developing coronary disease is up to four to five times higher, and stroke-related mortality is increased threefold in diabetics compared with non-diabetic individuals. The cardiovascular impact of diabetes is stronger in women than in men. Moreover, anginal pain may be absent in diabetic patients, leading to delayed recognition of angina pectoris and possible missed diagnosis of heart attack. The cardiovascular consequences of diabetes are related to both its specific metabolic effects and the potentiation of other risk factors such as obesity, dyslipidaemia, and hypertension, with which it is frequently associated in patients with type 2 diabetes. The association of diabetes with smoking is particularly harmful, and may mitigate the beneficial effects of successful control of other risk factors.

Management of diabetes

Insulin treatment is unavoidable for type 1 diabetes, but type 2 diabetes is frequently managed with a combination of diet, weight loss, and medications that work by potentiating the effects of insulin, although insulin injections may be necessary in resistant cases.

In patients with type 2 diabetes, the effects of good glucose control on primary and secondary cardiovascular prevention are difficult to isolate from, and are potentiated by, the mandatory tight control of the frequently coexistent risk factors hypertension, obesity, and dyslipidaemia. As a general rule, diabetic patients are considered at higher cardiovascular risk than non-diabetic individuals, and they are candidates for aggressive control of other risk factors even when these are present at borderline levels.

For more information on Diabetes, how it is diagnosed and the treatments available please see *Diabetes: The Facts* (information at the front of this book).

The concept of risk-factor profile and overall burden. When is specific treatment needed?

The upper limits of normal for BP, cholesterol, and blood sugar were mentioned in preceding sections. Higher values do not necessarily mean that treatment is immediately necessary, although follow-up and appropriate lifestyle changes are almost always recommended. Instead, the decision to start specific medication takes into account the overall cardiovascular risk or whether any one of the detected abnormalities is so severe that it justifies immediate treatment on its own. For example, borderline cholesterol will be specifically treated in a patient with coronary disease or concomitant risk factors, while mild hypercholesterolaemia may be just monitored in a healthy young woman without other risk factors. The overall cardiovascular risk is assessed using either tables and algorithms or dedicated software offered by medical organizations for the benefit of both patients and medical practitioners. Various national and international professional bodies may use slightly different measurements and strike a different balance between the relative weights of overall risk burden and the individual values of each measurable risk factor as an indication to initiate specific treatment.

The British Cardiac Society, the British Hypertension Society, the Stroke Association, and other specialized bodies agreed on common principles to define who should benefit from active risk factor reduction, and these are laid out in a common position document entitled *The Joint British Societies' Guidelines on Prevention Of Cardiovascular Disease In Clinical Practice* which was published in 2005.

According to this document, specific treatment for hypertension and hypercholesterolaemia is indicated for the following categories (see also Appendix A).

- Markedly elevated values (irrespective of the overall risk profile):
  - BP: ≥160/100 mmHg or evidence of target-organ damage
  - hypercholesterolaemia: total cholesterol/HDL-to-cholesterol ratio ≥6 or familial hypercholesterolaemia cases.
- Borderline or mildly elevated values:
  - overall estimated cardiovascular risk ≥20% over 10 years
  - diabetes
  - established atherosclerotic cardiovascular disease.

Even if specific drug therapy is not started, diet and lifestyle counselling are always recommended.

❓ Frequently Asked Questions

Q: Doctor, I am 55 years old and I am perfectly fit and healthy. Some of my friends started to take aspirin though they have no heart problems. I don't like taking medications that I don't need, but maybe, at my age, it would be sensible?

A: The decision whether to prescribe aspirin to asymptomatic individuals should be a balanced one. Aspirin is not totally without risk and age as such is not a reason to start taking aspirin. However, a combination of age and increased cardiovascular risk profile is accepted as a reasonable indication for low-dose (75 mg/day) aspirin. Your GP can discuss this with you and he/she will probably use a scoring system to assess your cardiovascular risk. The last UK guidelines recommend aspirin, in the absence of contraindications, for individuals more than 50 years old with an estimated cardiovascular risk of ≥20% over 10 years. The US guidelines are more liberal and suggest aspirin at a cardiovascular risk of ≥10% over 10 years.

Q: I've heard from many that occasionally drinking some wine may decrease the risk of heart disease. Is this true? What is a safe amount? Also, personally I enjoy beer and whisky as well. Are they also 'good' to prevent heart disease?

A: Existing data suggest that moderate alcohol consumption (≤3 units/day for men, ≤2 units/day for women) is associated with decreased coronary disease mortality. So, if you have no other contraindications and you don't see yourself at risk of addiction, you may enjoy alcohol in moderate amounts and possibly benefit from some cardiac protective effects. Although some data refer mainly to wine, there is no clear evidence of its superiority compared with other alcoholic beverages. Existing guidelines acknowledge the potential favourable effect of moderate alcohol use but stop short of recommending it as part of the primary prevention strategy for preventing coronary disease.

5

Atherosclerosis (Obstruction of the arteries)

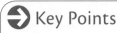 Key Points

- Atherosclerosis is more likely to develop and advance in the presence of so-called risk factors.

- Fat-related compounds and inflammatory tissue can accumulate on the inner surface of arteries and disrupt the vessels wall structure. This process is generally known as **atherosclerosis**.

- In advanced stages, atherosclerotic changes can result in vascular obstruction.

Blood vessels and atherosclerosis

The arteries are elastic smooth-walled vessels able to dilate to accommodate an increased blood flow as necessary during exercise. The artery wall has three concentric layers: the adventitia, a thin fibrotic external envelope; the media, a thick muscular layer; and the intima or endothelium, a thin inner layer whose cells synthesize various biologically important substances involved in vessel dilatation and blood clotting (Fig. 5.1). From at a very young age, cholesterol may accumulate in the arterial wall, beneath the intima, leading to so-called fatty streaks, which are found even in children and teenagers. This is the first stage of atherosclerosis, a process of hardening of the arteries due to fat accumulation (from Greek, *athera*: wax, because of the 'wax-like' appearance of fat accumulated in the vessel wall, and sclerosis: hardening). The atherosclerotic process is much more complex than the mere accumulation of fat, and involves an inflammatory reaction of the arterial wall, the net result of which is the development of the atherosclerotic plaque, which is the second stage of atherosclerosis. The typical atherosclerotic plaque has a core of cholesterol and inflammatory and degenerated cells (the atheroma) and an outer fibrous capsule. This fibrous plaque can remain stable or can slowly expand until the lumen of the vessel is partially or totally obstructed (Fig. 5.2) and symptoms develop. The arteries that are mainly involved are the coronary arteries, the neck arteries (carotid), the aorta, and the lower-limb arteries. Although atherosclerosis can occur in any individual, it is more frequent in those with risk factors. The association between risk factors and atherosclerosis is more evident in the young.

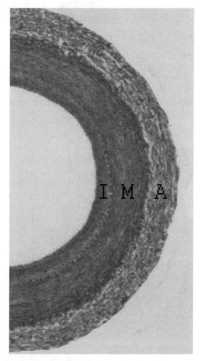

Figure 5.1 Microscopic section through an artery, demonstrating its trilayered structure: A, adventitia; I, intima; M, media.

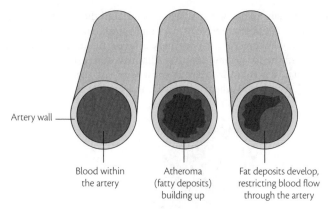

Artery wall —

Blood within
the artery

Atheroma
(fatty deposits)
building up

Fat deposits develop,
restricting blood flow
through the artery

Figure 5.2 Schematic representation of the stages of atherosclerosis. The apparently normal vessel wall can already be affected by fatty streaks.

(Reproduced with the kind permission of the British Heart Foundation, the copyright owner)

Types of heart disease and other problems

6

Coronary artery disease (ischaemic heart disease)

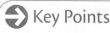 **Key Points**

- Coronary artery disease (CAD), resulting from narrowing of the coronary arteries, is the most common form of heart disease in adults.

- CAD manifests as a typical pain perceived during exercise: angina pectoris (AP).

- At times, there can be sudden complete occlusion of a coronary artery, inducing a heart attack: myocardial infarction (MI).

- A less common but devastating form of coronary artery disease is sudden cardiac death.

Ischaemic heart disease (IHD) and coronary artery disease (CAD) are two common names used interchangeably to describe the same condition: atherosclerotic (i.e. fatty) narrowing of the heart arteries with subsequent inadequate blood supply to the myocardium. CAD represents a major health problem in the Western world as it is responsible for heart attacks, angina pectoris (AP), heart failure, and the majority of cases of sudden death in middle-aged and elderly individuals.

Mechanisms

As a result of vessel narrowing, part of the cardiac muscle may not receive enough oxygen-enriched blood. There are two patterns of behaviour for the atherosclerotic plaque, with implications for the clinical presentation of CAD.

- **Stable plaque** The plaque is slowly growing, causing a gradual reduction of the arterial internal conduct cavity (lumen). This is initially corrected by compensatory dilatation of the vessel, but when the lumen is more than 75% obstructed, the artery cannot supply the necessary increase in blood flow during physical activities and the patient may experience anginal symptoms, such as pain or shortness of breath. The more severe the obstruction, the more likely the angina is to occur at lower levels of exercise. On the other hand, severe obstructions are related to slowly developing plaques whose lipid core is well contained in a fibrotic layer, and therefore they are less likely to rupture and cause acute coronary syndromes (see below).

♦ **Unstable plaque** 'Fresh' younger plaques are not obstructive enough to cause symptoms and are more likely to regress with cholesterol-lowering treatment. The downside is that their fat-rich core is more fluid and covered by a thinner capsule, so that they are more likely to bleed and suddenly increase in size or to fissure and promote local inflammation or clot formation that may further and acutely obstruct the vessel. This is the mechanism for suddenly worsening angina and myocardial infarction (MI). This is an apparent paradox, since the more severe plaques, associated with severe symptoms, are less likely to produce acute complications, while less severe asymptomatic plaques are responsible for most acute complications, possibly without any warning signs. To emphasize their common mechanism, both worsening (unstable) angina and MI are classified together as acute coronary syndromes. Cholesterol reduction has been shown to stop plaque progression and stabilize them.

Angina pectoris

There are few complaints that evoke such anguish and fear as chest pain or shortness of breath. AP is diagnosed when a patient reports a typical pain, generally associated with exercise. It reflects transient insufficient blood supply to the cardiac muscle because of narrowed coronary arteries, and is perceived as a typical pain. William Heberden, an English physician, first described its classical symptoms in the eighteenth century, and his clinical description remains valid today. In typical cases the patient experiences a painful pressure, heaviness, or burning feeling in the mid-chest area, with possible irradiation to the arms, neck or shoulders. This is typically triggered by exercise, but may be worsened or even elicited by other factors, such as exposure to cold, emotional stress, or a heavy meal. An anginal attack usually lasts from a few minutes to up to half an hour and is relieved by rest and/or use of short-acting nitrates such as nitroglycerine. A pain lasting just a few seconds is very unlikely to be anginal, and a pain lasting more than half an hour is more likely to be either non-cardiac or to represent a possible heart attack. A practical synopsis of anginal pain characteristics is provided on p. 10.

However, remember that there are many non-cardiac conditions that can mimic anginal pain, and that anginal pain presentation can also be highly atypical and different from the above description. Therefore only your physician can correctly diagnose the symptoms and differentiate between non-cardiac pain, angina, and heart attack.

Clinical presentations of angina

Stable exertional angina

This definition relates to the predictable occurrence of typical angina at the same level of exercise, which is frequently known by the patient who eventually changes his/her physical activity level, as needed, to avoid symptoms. This kind of angina is generally associated with a stable coronary plaque.

Unstable angina

This is a term generally used to describe either rapid worsening of pre-existing angina (more frequent or more severe attacks, occurrence at lower levels of exercise) or recent onset of angina, irrespective of its severity. The various patterns of unstable angina are a form of acute coronary syndrome and are related to an unstable plaque. They are treated more aggressively, frequently as an inpatient case, since they may herald a heart attack.

Equivalent angina

Occasional patients will experience shortness of breath or unusual fatigue, but no pain, with exercise. These symptoms may have the same significance as the typical painful angina. In these cases the diagnosis should be based on clinical suspicion, confirmatory tests, and ruling out other causes.

Atypical angina

This description is used to define patients who exhibit a mixture of typical and atypical features, i.e. the pain description is not typical (localization, character, duration) but the relationship to exercise is convincing, or the pain does sound anginal but is not related to exercise. These cases are relatively common and may pose a diagnostic challenge. As for equivalent angina, clinical suspicion and confirmatory tests are needed to establish the diagnosis.

Variant angina

This is also known as vasospastic or Prinzmetal angina after the cardiologist who first described it in 1959. It is a rare form of angina which is due mainly to transient spasm of the coronary arteries. Some cases characteristically occur in the early morning hours, but this is an unusual clinical presentation. Initially described in patients with normal coronary arteries, it may also be associated with coronary atherosclerosis, and some forms of atypical angina occurring at rest may be due to a vasospastic mechanism.

Medical treatment for angina (see also Chapter 12)

This typically includes statins to slow plaque progression, aspirin to help stabilize the plaque, nitrates or similar drugs to dilate the coronary arteries and prevent anginal attacks, and beta-blockers to prevent heart rate rise during exercise. You will also be give nitroglycerin tablets or spray to use when you have an anginal attack. In selected cases an angiography is performed in order to define the anatomy of the coronary vessels and to decide if a balloon dilatation or bypass surgery are indicated.

Revascularization treatment for angina

The term 'revascularization' refers to restoration of blood flow to an area of the heart muscle that is supplied by an obstructed coronary artery. This can be done either by dilating the narrowed artery using various procedures collectively known as percutaneous coronary intervention (PCI) or by a coronary artery bypass graft (CABG) surgical operation. Whether a patient with angina is managed only by medication, as described above, or with revascularization is an individualized decision. Except for well-selected cases, revascularization is not superior to drug treatment for prevention of a heart attack or cardiac death, but may be better for alleviating symptoms. The following are considered indications for revascularization rather than medical management:

◆ angina severe enough to interfere with usual activities and quality of life, despite optimal treatment

◆ involvement of 'strategic' segments of the coronary arteries, such as proximal vessels or the main left coronary artery

◆ evidence of severe and extensive ischaemia using tests such as stress echocardiography or nuclear perfusion tests.

Both options, i.e. medical treatment and revascularization, are valid for patients who do not satisfy these criteria and should be discussed (Table 6.1). Some patients may decide that their angina is not too limiting, so that they would rather continue with medication only than take the small risk related to the intervention. In a different scenario, the indication for revascularization does exist, but your doctor decides that in your particular case the risks of the procedure outweigh the benefits. This may be the case if your coronary disease is extensive and complex or because of coexisting problems such as renal failure, stroke, or general frailty.

Table 6.1 Relative advantages and drawbacks of a medical versus revascularization strategy in the management of patients with angina

Impact	Procedure
Symptom relief	Revascularization: frequently better than medical treatment
Need for continuous treatment	Some medications may be stopped after a successful revascularization
Prevention of heart attack or cardiac death	No difference
Procedure risk	Small risks for revascularization procedure

Percutaneous coronary intervention (PCI) procedures

Currently, PCI procedures are used in about a third of patients with coronary disease and have a major role in the emergency treatment of patients with heart attacks (see below). Until the early 1980s, CABG surgery was the only revascularization option for CAD patients. While very effective, this is a major open-chest surgical intervention, and it was felt that the risks were not worth taking in cases of non-critical coronary branch disease, even if the patient's angina was not fully controlled with medical treatment.

Percutaneous transluminal coronary angioplasty (PTCA)

Things started to change after a Swiss cardiologist, Andreas Gruntzig, successfully used a catheter-mounted balloon to dilate an obstructed coronary artery in a young patient in 1977. The technical concept behind the procedure is very straightforward. Catheter techniques are used to advance a specially designed balloon over a guide-wire in the diseased artery. At the site of obstruction the balloon is inflated, using a water solution, so that the atherosclerotic plaque is crushed and lumen patency is restored. Following this, the balloon is deflated and withdrawn from the artery (Figure 6.1). The procedure, called at the time percutaneous transluminal coronary angioplasty (PTCA), was rapidly accepted and soon, with continuous technological and balloon design advances, more patients with coronary disease had revascularization by PTCA rather then by CABG.

The immediate results were very good with a high success rate and a low rate of complications. Nevertheless, acute closure of the vessel was reported in about 5% of cases, occasionally necessitating emergency CABG. The technique was also adopted by other vascular specialties, being used to open carotic and peripheral arteries as well. Despite the initial enthusiasm and real contribution to the non-surgical management of these patients, it was soon found that the long-term results were less impressive, with up to 40% of successfully dilated lesions narrowing again (a process known as re-stenosis), so that some of the patients ended up having repeat procedures or being referred for CABG.

Re-stenosis is due to recoil of the dilated vessel and an inflammatory proliferative reaction of the vascular endothelium at the site of the dilatation. It is more likely to occur following dilatation of complex lesions. Both re-stenosis and the risk of acute occlusion were addressed by a further development—the use of special devices called stents.

Stents

Stents, which were introduced in the late 1980s, are ingeniously designed small mesh- or coil-like cylinders, generally mounted on a balloon, which scaffold the artery after dilatation and thus avoid the need for emergency CABG in the rare cases of acute artery occlusion. They were expected to significantly reduce

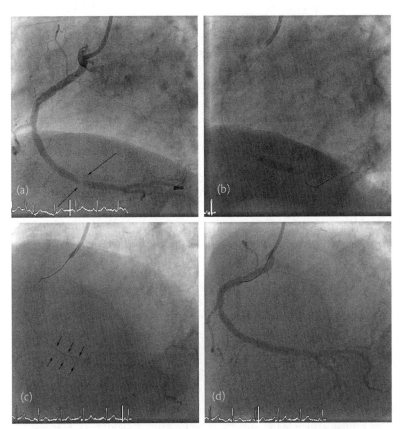

Figure 6.1 Balloon opening and stenting of a stenotic coronary artery: (a) diagnostic injection showing a tight lesion in the right coronary artery (long arrows); (b) the balloon is advanced over a wire and inflated at the site of the lesion; (c) the stent is now deployed and faintly visualized in the arterial lumen (short arrows); (d) final results, showing a patent coronary artery.

re-stenosis as well, but while re-stenosis rates were indeed lowered compared with standard PTCA, they remained high enough (10–20%) to be of concern. The long-term risk of re-stenosis was further reduced by the introduction of a new generation of stents, called drug-eluting stents (DESs) as opposed to the previous bare metal stents (BMSs). DESs are impregnated with an immunosuppressive drug that is slowly released to inhibit the wall thickening responsible for long-term re-stenosis. Indeed, re-stenosis occurs in less than 10% of cases after DES use, i.e. four-times less than after standard PTCA without stents.

Atherectomy

Another PCI technique, which is less frequently used, is atherectomy in which a hard atherosclerotic plaque is cut and 'shaved' with a special device.

Summary of PCI techniques

The vast majority of PCIs are stenting procedures, with DESs used in more than half of the cases. Currently, the immediate success rate is over 90%, with a risk of death or major heart attack of less than 1%. The use of stents, and especially DESs, slightly increases the risk of late clot formation within the stent because of the thrombogenic effect of this foreign body in contact with the blood flow. This rare but possible complication is effectively prevented by the use of a more aggressive anti-platelet regimen that includes both aspirin and clopidogrel (see pp. 106-108 to be taken for extended periods of time, possibly a year or more for DESs.

What happens after PCI?

Following an elective procedure and in the absence of complications, you should expect to leave the hospital the next day and return to your normal activities within a few days. Your usual medications may be altered: the treatment you receive for risk factors will remain the same and clopidogrel (Plavix) will be added to your aspirin, but nitrates and beta-blockers may be reduced or stopped altogether, depending on the particularities of your case. If the main reason for the procedure was angina, you should notice a significant improvement or disappearance of symptoms altogether. You should contact your doctor if your angina persists, if new symptoms appear, or if there is progressive swelling, pain, or more than a mild bruising at the site of the intervention (groin, wrist).

Coronary artery bypass graft (CABG) surgery

The principle for CABG surgery is technically straightforward: it implies bypassing the obstructed (or 'occluded') coronary segment using a vascular graft which has one extremity connected to the aortic root and the other to the occluded artery beyond the narrowed site. The technique was pioneered in the late 1960s by the Argentinean surgeon Rene Favaloro and, until the advent of PCI, it was the only available revascularization technique for patients with severe angina or high-risk disease features. Technically, this is an open-chest but not an open-heart intervention, performed under general anaesthesia and lasting for a few hours. Either lower-limb veins (saphenous veins grafts) or arterial conduits such as the internal mammary artery (running behind the chest wall) or an upper-limb artery (radial artery) are used to bypass the obstructed segment (Figure 6.2). Like PCI procedures, CABG does not cure the atherosclerotic disease of your vessels, but it is very effective in restoring blood supply and relieving anginal symptoms. In simple cases in otherwise healthy individuals, the operative mortality is 1% or less, and in the absence of complications you should expect to leave the hospital within a week.

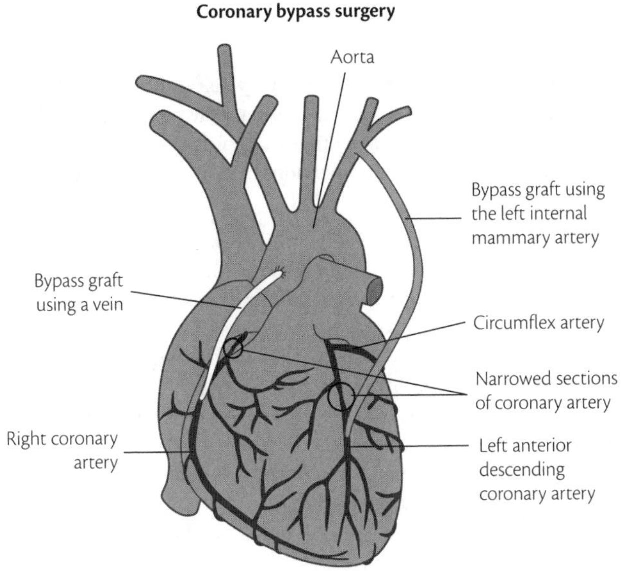

Coronary bypass surgery

Figure 6.2 Schematic representation of typical coronary artery bypass surgery. In this case the left internal mammary artery is used to bypass stenosis in the left anterior descending artery, and a venous graft is used to bypass a stenosis in the right coronary artery.

(Reproduced with the kind permission of the British Heart Foundation, the copyright owner)

What happens after CABG?

As for PCI procedures, if angina was the main indication for surgery you should experience immediate relief, and your medications may be altered as described above. However, the overall recovery period is longer, and in some cases it may take a few months for you to reach a full and unimpeded level of activity. This is very variable, and depends on your age, coexistent diseases, and any complications that may have occurred during or immediately after the operation. Engaging in a cardiac rehabilitation programme can be very useful and shortens the recovery period, and most institutions offer rehabilitation to their patients after surgery. Some patients remain anaemic and this may contribute to general fatigue, but this complication is easily identified and treated. Also, the healing process of the central chest bone (sternum) may take time; this, combined with damage to some nerve endings, explains some persistent chest pains that may take time to resolve and are managed with usual painkillers. These pains are different from your usual anginal pains, and usually you should have no difficulty in differentiating between the two. If in doubt, consult your doctor.

Frequently Asked Question

Q: Last year I underwent coronary artery bypass graft surgery. The operation was a success and now I have no angina, play tennis, and feel as 'good as new'. Also, the doctors told me that there was no damage to my heart. Do I still need to take all my medications? I hoped that I could get rid of most of them.

A: You'll probably be able to get rid of some of them but others will have to be continued. If you were taking nitrates for angina relief, there is no reason to continue now that you are symptom free. On the other hand, any medication that you were taking to control risk factors (i.e. for hypertension, hypercholesterolaemia, diabetes) should be continued, if appropriate, to prevent further atherosclerotic lesions. Aspirin is also practically 'for life' in your case. Therefore one aspirin tablet is the minimum that you should take; beyond that it depends on your risk-factor profile, although most practitioners would probably continue a statin as well even if your cholesterol levels are in the normal range.

CABG or PCI?

In view of its obvious convenience and advantages, such as avoidance of major surgery and general anaesthesia, short hospital stay, good results, and low complication rates, PCI is by far the most frequently used revascularization procedure today. CABG remains the procedure of choice in cases of:

- multiple narrowings involving multiple coronary arteries
- lesions that are technically difficult to tackle with PCI
- selected patients with diabetes
- need for concomitant non-coronary intervention, such as valve surgery.

As a rule, in technically difficult cases long-term results tend to be better with CABG than with PCI, especially if arterial grafts are used. In cases that do not have a straightforward indication for either PCI or CABG, the decision is taken after an in-depth discussion between you and your cardiologist about the advantages and disadvantages of each method in your particular case.

Myocardial infarction (heart attack)

A sudden obstruction of a coronary artery, usually by a clot, will deprive an area of the cardiac muscle of its blood supply. This is what is called a myocardial infarction (MI), but is frequently referred to as a heart attack. If the obstruction of the artery is complete, the affected ventricular wall will be completely (full-thickness) infarcted, i.e. myocardial cells will eventually die and be replaced by scar tissue; if the obstruction is partial only, or if other branches supply the same territory, the infarction will be more patchy and will not necessarily affect the whole thickness of the ventricular wall. The former condition is frequently associated with a typical ECG appearance (ST-segment elevation) (Figure 6.3), and therefore it is called ST-elevation myocardial infarction (STEMI). The latter does not generally exhibit ST elevation and therefore is referred to as non-ST-elevation myocardial infarction (NSTEMI). If the blood supply is not re-established quickly (within a few hours) by either balloon dilatation or clot-dissolving (thrombolytic) drugs, permanent damage with scarring of the cardiac muscle occurs. Most improvements in acute MI by restoring blood flow through an occluded artery relate to patients with STEMI.

Why does myocardial infarction happen?

Most cases of MI occur in patients with atherosclerotic coronary artery disease, but, as opposed to anginal attacks that are typically triggered by exertion, there is no immediate cause for a MI and, in fact, most cases occur at rest without any identifiable trigger. However, we do know that heart attacks are related to unstable non-obstructive coronary plaques which may bleed and increase their size or fissure and be covered by a thrombus (Figure 6.4), although

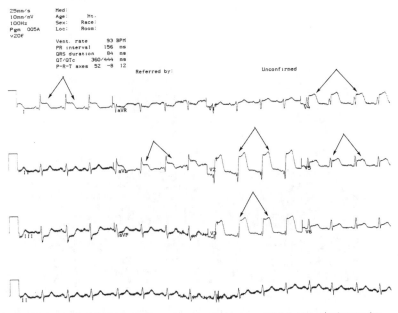

Figure 6.3 Typical ECG in a patient presenting with a large STEMI. Note the impressive shift upwards of the ST segment (arrows) compared with the normal ECG in Figure 3.6.

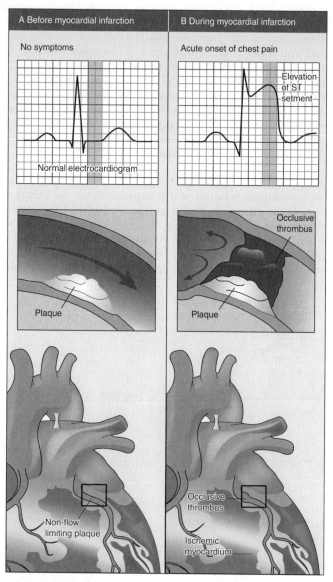

Figure 6.4 Sequence of events in a coronary artery with pre-existent coronary disease, resulting in an acute STEMI, and the beneficial effect of primary PCI. The non-obstructive and possibly asymptomatic plaque (a) becomes unstable and (b) is covered by an acute clot that completely occludes the artery, causing an acute MI.

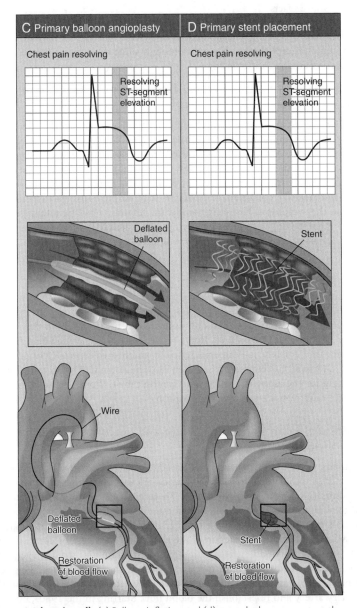

Figure 6.4 (*continued*) (c) Balloon inflation and (d) stent deployment restore the blood flow and abort the evolution of the MI, minimizing the myocardial damage.

Reproduced from Keeley EC, Hillis LD (2007). Primary PCI for myocardial infarction with ST-segment elevation. *New England Journal of Medicine* **356**: 47–54, with permission.

why this happens at a given moment is less clear. The patient may be totally asymptomatic until the acute event, although some do notice a worsening of pre-existing angina (unstable angina).

What are the symptoms? When should I suspect that I have a heart attack?

When severe angina-like pain unrelated to physical activity occurs and lasts for more than half an hour, with no or minimal relief after nitroglycerin (GTN), MI is suspected. Associated shortness of breath, sweating, nausea, and weakness strengthen the diagnosis. However, the clinical presentation may be highly variable, ranging from a severe form of these typical symptoms to some light or upset-stomach-like condition, and patients without previous heart disease may misread the symptoms. Not infrequently, the infarction can be totally painless or accompanied only by some vague symptoms (silent MI) and recognized only later because of an abnormal ECG or complications.

What should I do if I suspect that I may have had a heart attack?

Time is essential in providing optimum treatment. If you think that you may be having a heart attack, don't be concerned that it may be a false alarm. Immediately call the emergency or ambulance service (999 in the UK, 112 in all EC countries) and then sit or lie down and try to rest while waiting for the ambulance. Chew an aspirin tablet, if one is readily available, even if you are already taking aspirin.

Myocardial infarction management and outcome: a historical perspective

For many years the management of an acute MI was based on observation, rest, and symptom relief only. A major landmark was the setting up of coronary care units (CCUs) in the early 1960s. These allowed continuous monitoring and treatment of life-threatening arrhythmias during the critical first 3–5 days and thus significantly reduced the number of deaths. However, the mechanism of a MI, i.e. the acute obstruction of the artery and the need for early opening of the vessel and blood flow restoration in order to minimize the damage to the heart, was not addressed until the late 1970s. At that time, drugs like streptokinase (STK) or similar substances were shown to break up the clot in the coronary artery and re-establish the blood flow. Starting in the 1980s, opening the obstructed artery with 'clot-busting' drugs such as STK became the norm for STEMIs (there were no benefits of thrombolysis for NSTEMIs), and this treatment, known as thrombolysis or fibrinolysis, brought a further decrease in mortality after a heart attack. However, thrombolytic drugs are only able to open the artery in 50–60% of cases, and the success rate may be even lower with late presentation. Also, up to a quarter of patients presenting with acute MI are not given thrombolysis because of concerns about bleeding complications. Beginning in the 1990s, PCI techniques were extended to emergency opening of the occluded artery in patients with STEMI, an approach known as primary PCI (Figure 6.4). Immediate and long-term results are better with primary PCI, which has tended to become the preferred treatment, although fibrinolysis is still widely used in many places. The use of either primary PCI or fibrinolysis (collectively known as reperfusion therapy) together with CCU monitoring for the first few days and standard use of drugs such as statins, beta-blockers, and ACE inhibitors has resulted in a dramatic decrease in mortality due to acute MI, with reported mortality rates as low as 5–7% and a very good chance of returning to a normal life.

What happens when I reach the hospital?

Hospitalization is always necessary for MI and in uncomplicated cases will last for about a week or less. Some measures will be taken almost automatically, either in the ambulance or immediately on arrival:

- being given oxygen
- being given an aspirin to chew,
- being given drugs for pain,
- taking blood
- establishing venous access.

There will be quite a lot of activity around you, involving nurses and medical staff. This should not worry you; it just shows that good routines are being followed. An ECG will help decide whether this is indeed a heart attack and whether you should benefit from reperfusion treatment. If you are deemed suitable for reperfusion, you will either be given a 'clot-busting' drug or prepared for primary PCI, depending on local facilities. Again depending on local set-up and routines, this decision may be taken by the ambulance team, and, if appropriate, you may be taken directly to the catheterization suite. Following either the primary PCI or the administration of the fibrinolytic drug, there is a good chance that you will feel better, and you will be taken to the coronary care unit for monitoring. A few drugs that are practically a standard package after a heart attack would have been started by now:

- aspirin and clopidogrel to help maintain the artery open
- statins in high doses to lower the cholesterol and help reduce the inflammation of the coronary artery wall
- beta-blockers to prevent arrhythmias
- ACE inhibitors to minimize the effect of the heart attack on the cardiac muscle.

In the absence of complications you can expect to leave the CCU for the regular cardiology ward after about 3 days and to be discharged home within a week. If an angiogram had not been performed on admission, you may have one before discharge, depending on your overall condition and the results of tests such as an exercise test and an echo scan.

What happens after I go home?

Following a heart attack you will be discharged from the hospital when your condition is considered stable and you have undergone all the tests and procedures deemed necessary. As mentioned above, in uncomplicated cases this should happen within a week or even less, and in fact the great majority of patients return to a normal life after a heart attack. When going home, you should expect to be informed about:

- the final assessment of your heart condition
- the medications that you have to take and for how long
- scheduled follow-up appointment in the outpatients clinic
- pace of resuming normal activities
- expected timing of return to work and any possible limitations
- practical advice on driving, flying, or resuming sexual activities.

In most cases, you will also start a rehabilitation scheme that includes both counselling and enrolment in a well-titrated physical fitness programme. While this may not be mandatory, especially after small uncomplicated heart attacks, it is extremely useful for guiding and helping your 'return to normal', giving you feedback on the progress you are making in increasing your activity level, and monitoring your adherence to all recommendations that you received on discharge. Most patients engaged in a rehabilitation programme report a very positive experience, and there is a large body of evidence that supports the beneficial role of rehabilitation programmes to shorten the recovery period and hasten return to normal activity levels after a heart attack.

 Frequently Asked Question

Q: I occasionally have to use nitroglycerin spray. Of late I have noticed that it takes a longer time until the pain goes away. How many times can I use it? Is there any danger if I use it a few times?

A: When used as a spray or as sublingual tablets, nitroglycerin is a rapidly acting drug. Therefore it can be repeated at 5-minute intervals without the risk of overdosage. However, persistent or rapidly recurrent pain may signal that this is more than your usual angina attack. It is generally recommended that you should seek medical attention if more than three doses are needed.

Q: I had a heart attack last month but now I am practically back to normal. My wife is thinking of taking a nice relaxing vacation. What is the earliest time that I can embark on air travel?

A: There are few data on the safety of flying soon after a heart attack, but the overall tolerance is good and a consensus exists that it is safe to fly about 2–3 weeks after an uncomplicated heart attack, provided that your clinical condition is stable and you can perform usual activities without limitation. You should consult your GP or cardiologist and make sure that there are no limitations in your travel medical insurance or due to flight company regulations.

Q: I am 55 years old and I had a heart attack last month. Except for the first 2 days I felt reasonably well during my hospital stay, but my cardiologist informed me that this was quite a big heart attack and there was some damage to the heart muscle. I also had two stents fit into the arteries of the heart. I take quite a lot of medications but overall I feel well and fit now and I have resumed most of my usual activities. I am not confident about sex though. Are there any dangers? Should I be careful about anything in particular?

A: As a general rule, sex is safe after a heart attack, once you feel well and able to perform regular activities. In fact, less than 1% of myocardial infarctions occur during a sexual act. From the point of view of effort intensity, you can think of sexual activity as a moderate effort, such as a brisk 20-minute walk. Most authorities agree that sexual activity can be resumed a few weeks after a heart attack if your condition has stabilized and you are comfortable with moderate levels of exercise, as described above. Depending on the particulars of your case, your doctor may refer you for an exercise test, to assess, among other things, your fitness for increased levels of effort. Common sense dictates that sexual activity should be resumed gradually, and at the beginning you should 'test' yourself and see how you respond. Using less demanding love-making techniques, such as having your partner above you, is a reasonable approach. If angina, shortness of breath, or dizziness occur, you should refrain from further activities and consult your doctor.

Besides 'safety' concerns, sexual dysfunction is also a possible issue after a heart attack and generally in cardiac patients. Some elements of sexual dysfunction may predate the heart attack and may be exacerbated by the psychological impact of the cardiac event, performance anxiety on resuming sexual activities, coexistent pathologies such as diabetes, or the use of certain drugs such as beta-blockers. Viagra can be used, although caution is advised in those with borderline low blood pressure or taking nitrates, in which case the concomitant use of Viagra is contraindicated. In these cases a frank discussion with your doctor and the rehabilitation team is necessary.

7

Rhythm disturbances (Arrhythmia)

→ Key Points

- The normal resting heat rate in adults varies between 60 and 90 beats/minute.

- Extrasystolae or premature beats are isolated 'out of rhythm' beats that occur with varying frequency.

- Arrhythmias and rapid (tachycardia) or slow (bradycardia) heart rhythm are a relatively common occurrence.

- Flutter and fibrillation refer to more complex and prolonged irregular heart beats.

- The presence of a rhythm disturbance does not necessarily mean an organic heart disease is present, although some investigations may be necessary.

- Specific treatment is not always needed.

Extrasystolae

Extrasystolae are isolated irregular beats, of either ventricular or atrial origin, frequently followed by a short slowing of the heart rate (Figure 7.1). Extrasystolae may occur with variable frequency, ranging from a few isolated ones to thousands within 24 hours. Occasionally, triggers such as excessive coffee or alcohol drinking or emotional stress are present, but in most cases there is no immediate reason for occurrence.

They tend to be more frequent with advanced age or on the background of heart disease, but may also be encountered in youngsters and without any underlying heart disease. Extrasystolae may be completely asymptomatic or be unpleasantly perceived as a strong unexpected heart beat or a thumping feeling in the throat, or the subsequent heart slowing may be perceived as a worrying stillness of the heart. Occasionally, the presence of extrasystolae prompts further tests to rule out a previously unrecognized heart condition, but frequently, especially in

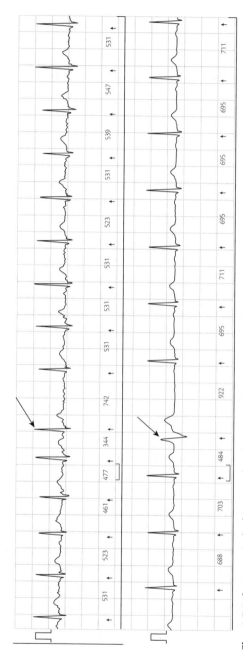

Figure 7.1 Supraventricular (upper row) and ventricular (lower row) extrasystolae (arrows) detected by Holter monitoring in a healthy individual complaining of rare palpitations. Both extrasystolae have an early occurrence and are followed by a slight pause, but the ventricular one has a different morphology from baseline rhythm.

young people, they are a benign arrhythmia and all that is needed is reassurance without specific treatment, although beta-blockers may be helpful.

Tachycardia and tachyarrhythmias

Tachycardia is defined in adults as a heart rhythm of over 100 beats/minute occurring at rest. Depending on whether it is regular or irregular and on its ECG appearance, tachycardia may represent just an increased activity of the sinus node activity (sinus tachycardia) or a proper arrhythmia.

Sinus tachycardia

Sinus tachycardia is the acceleration of the normal heart rhythm. The ECG of a patient with isolated sinus tachycardia may be otherwise completely normal and only show a high heart rate. Although it is frequently a concern for the patient or a reason for referral to a cardiology consultation, isolated sinus tachycardia is very rarely due to cardiac disease, and is more likely to be situational (emotion, psychological stress) or reflect a non-cardiac disease, such as:

◆ anaemia

◆ hyperthyroidism

◆ diabetes

◆ painful conditions

◆ fever.

Sinus tachycardia can be lowered with beta-blockers, but this is not generally necessary; rather, the underlying condition should be identified and managed appropriately.

Postural tachycardia syndrome (POTS)

Some individuals may have an abnormal heart rate increase while standing. In more severe forms, it is experienced as unpleasant pounding of the heart and head, and may also be accompanied by a drop in blood pressure. POTS is an uncommon condition (although mild cases are probably not diagnosed) which is more frequent in women. In some cases, a neurological problem is present, but commonly no cause can be identified. The treatment is based mainly on avoiding dehydration, exercise training, and reconditioning, although specific medications may be used in refractory cases.

Atrial fibrillation and flutter

Atrial fibrillation (AF) and atrial flutter (AFl) are two supraventricular arrhythmias with different electric mechanisms but similar clinical features. In AF, the electrical activity of the atria is totally disorganized, with the ventricles being activated in a random way, resulting in an irregular and generally fast heart rate. In AFl, the electrical activity of the atria is regular and rapid, resulting in a fast and usually regular heart rate. Both AF and AFl are associated with pre-existent organic heart disease or hypertension and their prevalence increases with age, being quite frequent in the elderly (up to 9% in octogenarians), in whom they may occur without an identifiable cause. Rarely, AF and AFl may be encountered in otherwise young healthy individuals, although this is unusual. Occasionally, they may be related to hyperthyroidism (of which they may be the first manifestation) or an acute non-cardiac disease, or binge drinking. The symptoms, clinical presentation, complications, and management of both conditions are very similar.

Symptoms

Both AF and AFl may occur repeatedly for short (hours to days) periods of time and resolve spontaneously (paroxysmal AF/AFl) or may be permanent (chronic AF/AFl). Patients with AF/AFl may be totally asymptomatic and have the arrhythmia discovered on a routine examination. More commonly, however, they will notice a strong, rapid, and irregular heart beat.

If the arrhythmia is long lasting, fatigue, shortness of breath, and a general picture of heart failure may develop, especially in the elderly and those with pre-existing heart disease. In fact, it is not unusual for some of these patients not to notice the irregularity of their pulse and to seek medical attention for the above symptoms, at which time the arrhythmia is found.

Complications

Heart failure

Heart failure symptoms in some patients with AF/AFl may be related not only to the abnormal rhythm, but also to a real deterioration of the ventricular contractility due to long-standing high heart rates. If there is no background heart disease, the contractility of the 'tired' left ventricle is expected to recover once the heart rate is under control.

Thromboembolic complications

The atria of patients with AF, and to a certain extent of those with AFl, are not really contracting because of their abnormal electrical activation. As a result, the blood moves very slowly within the atrial cavity and this may promote clot formation. Occasionally, parts of the clot may detach and travel with the blood stream until they become lodged in a peripheral artery, resulting in a stroke or obstruction of limb arteries. This is a rare but potentially devastating complication. Fortunately, not all patients are at high risk, and this can be prevented, when appropriate, with chronic anticoagulation.

Management

There are two areas of management decisions for patients with AF/AFl.

Rhythm and rate management

Lowering the heart rate of AF/AFl patients is frequently the first step in their treatment. Rate control is usually achieved with drugs, such as beta-blockers, calcium-channel blockers, or digoxin, which will leave the heart rhythm irregular but with rates within normal limits. Patients with spontaneously or easily controlled rates, who are completely asymptomatic and have no functional limitation, may eventually be left in chronic well controlled AF/AFl. This approach, referred to as 'rate control strategy', has been shown to have good tolerance and outcome.

Reversing the arrhythmia to normal sinus rhythm (cardioversion) is referred to as 'rhythm control strategy' and is indicated when the AF/AFl is not well tolerated even with good rate control. Even patients who seem to tolerate their arrhythmia well are considered for rhythm control if they are young and active or if this is the first episode. In borderline cases, the best approach is decided taking into account background heart disease, concomitant diseases, general fitness, and likelihood of success.

Cardioversion

Cardioversion is an active act of reverting the fibrillation or flutter to a normal sinus rhythm. This is an in-hospital procedure and can be achieved using specific drugs (medical cardioversion) or by delivering an electric shock (electrical cardioversion).

Medical cardioversion

In well-tolerated cases of recent-onset AF, specific drugs (flecainide, propafenone, amiodarone, sotalol) are used, generally intravenously, to attempt to restore sinus rhythm. The overall success rate of medical cardioversion is highly variable (50–90%), but when successful this approach obviates the need for electrical cardioversion.

Electrical cardioversion

Electrical cardioversion, referred to as direct current cardioversion (DCC) is attempted when medical cardioversion is unsuccessful, when the patient's condition requires immediate restoration of sinus rhythm, or when it is considered to be the most appropriate approach as a first step.

How do I prepare for cardioversion?

Depending on the specifics of your case, DCC may be performed during the same hospitalization or you may be given an appointment for an elective procedure. If you are not already taking anticoagulants, DCC will generally be delayed to ensure that you have been taking anticoagulants for at least 3 weeks. Your cardiologist will also decide whether you should be 'loaded' with an anti-arrhythmic drug beforehand. Most medical institutions will provide you with an explanatory leaflet.

What happens on the day of cardioversion?

You will be instructed when and if to take your medications. Since DCC is performed under general anaesthesia, you will be kept fasting and you will be assessed by an anaesthetist. At the time of the procedure, you will be given a short-acting anaesthetic and when you are deeply asleep, an electric shock will be delivered to your chest using two paddles connected to a special machine (defibrillator). If the first shock is not successful, a few more may be tried with increasing levels of energy. You should wake up quickly and recover completely in a few hours. You should be informed about the outcome of the procedure, given instructions for medications and follow-up, and, in the absence of complications, you can expect to leave the hospital later the same day or the next day.

What are the odds of success?

The immediate success rate for DCC is very high, in the range of 90%. DCC is a widely used and time-tested procedure.

Are there any risks?

With good preparation, the odds for any significant complications are very low. There is a theoretical risk of stroke but, with good anticoagulation, the odds for this are 1% or less.

What happens after the procedure?

You will be instructed to continue your anticoagulation for at least 1 month. Depending on the specifics of your case, the odds of recurrence, and your thromboembolic risk, anticoagulation and anti-arrhythmic drugs may be prescribed for longer periods, occasionally indefinitely.

How are recurrences prevented?

After cardioversion, there may be no recurrence of the arrhythmia if this was the first episode and you are otherwise fit and healthy, with a normal heart. This is true especially if a clear triggering factor could be identified as the immediate reason for your arrhythmia. Otherwise, the risk of recurrence may be high, with more than 70% of patients relapsing into atrial fibrillation. A similar problem is faced by patients with repeated bouts of atrial fibrillation. The risk of recurrence can be significantly diminished, although not abolished, by using various anti-arrhythmic drugs. However, some of these drugs are contraindicated in certain forms of heart disease, and others may have significant side effects. An individualized decision should be taken in each case. For patients with poorly tolerated AF and incapacitating recurrences of AF/AFl, in whom anti-arrhythmic drugs are ineffective or not tolerated, catheter-based procedures are available to correct the electrical abnormality responsible for the fibrillation. During these procedures (atrial fibrillation ablation), multiple sites in the left atrium are 'burned' by delivery of radiofrequency energy so that circuits used by fibrillation waves are interrupted. The procedure-related risks are small and the overall success rate is 60–70%.

Thromboembolic risk management

A mentioned above, blood clots can develop in the fibrillating atrium and may be responsible for strokes, but this risk can be more than halved with the use of chronic anticoagulation, usually with warfarin. However, long-term warfarin use is not totally risk free either, with possible gastric or intracerebral bleeding. In addition, the risk of stroke varies greatly among AF/AFl patients. Therefore anticoagulation is not given automatically, but only if indicated in patients whose risk of stroke without anticoagulation is considered higher than the risk of bleeding with anticoagulation. The following are considered to increase the odds of stroke in patients with AF and are used in various scoring systems:

- advanced age
- arterial hypertension
- diabetes
- heart failure
- left ventricular systolic dysfunction
- mitral valve disease
- previous stroke.

The same criteria apply for both AF and AFl, and whether the arrhythmia is chronic or permanent. Patients undergoing cardioversion are anticoagulated for at least a month before and after the procedure, irrespective of their risk profile.

Paroxysmal supraventricular tachycardia (PSVT)

Regular tachycardias with heart rates above 200 beats/minute may occur when an abnormal fascicle of fibres, either within the AV node or in its vicinity, allows very fast conduction of the electric stimuli from the atria to the ventricles. Some of these cases belong to the Wolff–Parkinson–White syndrome, characterized by a typical ECG appearance of a short PR interval and a distorted QRS, but in most cases the ECG is completely normal except for the tachycardia paroxysms. In contrast with AF/AFl, PSVTs can occur at any age, including in children and teenagers, and are not generally associated with organic heart disease. There is no specific trigger for PSVT attacks and their occurrence is variable and unpredictable. Many paroxysms are short, cease spontaneously, and, except for an unpleasant heart beat, are well tolerated unless organic heart disease is present. Some patients may abort an attack by so-called vagal manoeuvres, such as stimulating the throat to induce gagging, holding the breath and trying to exhale against a closed mouth, or immersing the face in ice-cold water. Prolonged attacks of rapid PSVT become symptomatic, possibly inducing shortness of breath, dizziness, or chest pain. These cases have to be managed in hospital where intravenous drugs such as adenosine, verapamil, beta-blockers, or digoxin are used to abort the attack. However, prolonged hospitalization is not necessary in most cases.

PSVT management

Cases with rare, short-lasting, and well-tolerated attacks can be managed with observation only. Beta-blockers or calcium-channel blockers can be tried, but the results are variable. More specific anti-arrhythmic drugs are efficient, but long-term treatment may not be the best approach in otherwise active young individuals. Catheter-based ablation procedures are the best option for long-term results, with small risks and success rates above 95%.

Ventricular tachycardia (VT)

Ventricular tachycardia is a tachycardic heart rhythm of ventricular origin. The rhythm is regular, but the ECG appearance is generally very different from that of other rhythm disturbances. Although rare asymptomatic short runs are occasionally encountered in otherwise healthy individuals, VT is a potentially dangerous arrhythmia, frequently associated with either organic heart disease or a genetic predisposition.

VT in patients with decreased left ventricular function is a particularly high-risk condition. Short runs of VT may be well tolerated, but prolonged and rapid runs may result in severe symptoms, ranging from heart failure and dizziness to syncope or sudden death, and occasionally may need immediate interruption with an electric shock (Figure 7.2). The finding of VT, whether symptomatic or not, should prompt a comprehensive work-up for the underlying abnormality. Almost all patients with VT are evaluated with an echocardiographic scan. The use of other tests, such as angiography or MRI, depends on the particulars of each case. Low-risk cases may occasionally be managed with anti-arrhythmic drugs or beta-blockers, but high-risk cases benefit from an implantable defibrillator.

Ventricular fibrillation (VF)

This is a lethal arrhythmia characterized by a completely irregular electrical activity and contraction of the left ventricle, resulting in loss of mechanical activity. It may complicate a prolonged and rapid VT, or occur as such, mainly in association with a heart attack. The clinical picture is of loss of consciousness and cardiac arrest. Unless immediately recognized and interrupted with an electric shock, VF is invariably fatal.

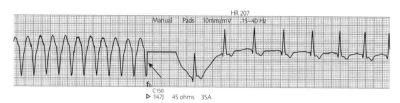

Figure 7.2 Rapid ventricular tachycardia, inducing hypotension. Normal rhythm is restored with an electric shock (arrow).

Bradycardia

Bradycardia is defined as a heart rate less than 60 beats/minute. Severe brady-cardia (less than 40 beats/minute) may be symptomatic, ranging in severity from mild dizziness to frank syncope. Bradycardia can occur because of either a slow-ing of the normal heart rate (sinus bradycardia) or a slowing of the conduction of the electrical impulses from the atria to the ventricles (atrioventricular block). As a rule, symptomatic bradycardias, not related to a reversible cause, have no effective drug treatment and are managed with permanent pacemakers.

Sinus bradycardia

Physiological sinus bradycardia

Mild sinus bradycardia is normal at night. Performance athletes frequently exhibit moderate bradycardia; however this is well tolerated, even in the 40-50 beats/minute range. Lack of symptoms and associated diseases, obvious back-ground, and good response of heart rhythm to exercise confirm the diagnosis of this finding as benign, in fact normal, and in no need of treatment or further investigation.

Abnormal sinus bradycardia

Drug-induced bradycardia

Mild bradycardia is frequently encountered in patients treated with beta-block-ers or some calcium-channel blockers, such as verapamil or diltiazem. In fact, a resting heart rate of 50–60 beats/minute in these patients may be considered a desirable target and an indicator of an effective dose. If well tolerated, it should not be a matter of concern or a reason to decrease the dose. However, acciden-tal or voluntary overdose or a combination of drugs may induce various degrees of moderate to severe bradycardia. Mild cases are managed with monitoring only, waiting for the drug to clear from the body. Cases of profound bradycardia may result in severe dizziness, syncope, and transient heart and renal failure due to decreased cardiac output. These patients are managed in cardiac care units and frequently need insertion of a temporary pacemaker to ensure an effective heart rate until the effects of the drug resolve.

Sick sinus syndrome

Degenerative changes in the sinus node can occur in an otherwise normal heart, resulting in progressive sinus bradycardia, sometimes alternating with periods of rapid arrhythmias. Mild cases need follow-up only, but the only effective management of advanced bradycardia and symptoms is a permanent pacemaker.

Atrioventricular block (AVB)

The heart rate can slow down not only as a result of sinus bradycardia, as detailed above, but also if the electrical impulses generated at atrial level are blocked and do not reach the ventricles. This condition is known as atrioventricular block (AVB). There are three degrees of AVB.

♦ First-degree AVB: the propagation of the electrical stimulus from the atria to the ventricle is only slowed down and not blocked. This condition is asymptomatic but is recognized on ECG, and in certain cases may warrant follow-up or caution when prescribing certain drugs.

♦ Second-degree AVB: the propagation of the electrical impulse from the atria to the ventricle is intermittently blocked, resulting in various degree of bradycardia. Some forms of second-degree AVB are benign and may even be present in athletes during sleep, while others are symptomatic or signal a possible evolution to more severe forms.

♦ Third-degree AVB: no atrial electrical impulse can reach the ventricle. An alternative focus usually takes over to maintain the heart rate, but if this safety mechanism fails (Figure 7.3), profound bradycardia and even complete cardiac arrest can ensue, resulting in syncope or death.

Some instances of AVB occur because of isolated degenerative changes in the electrical conduction system of the heart, while others are related to organic heart disease. Management is similar to that of other mechanisms of bradycardia, i.e. a pacemaker is required in advanced symptomatic cases or when the odds for progression to more severe forms are high.

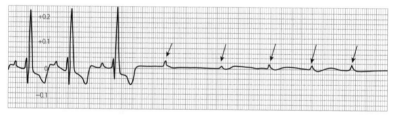

Figure 7.3 Sudden occurrence of complete atrioventricular block. The first three cardiac cycles are normal, but the subsequent P waves (arrows) are not followed by ventricular contractions, resulting in cardiac arrest.

8

Congestive heart failure

> ## ⟳ Key Points
>
> ◆ Cardiac failure is a condition characterized by typical symptoms of shortness of breath, fatigue, and evidence of fluid retention. It is less of a disease on its own but rather the end-result of other diseases such as coronary artery disease, valvular disease, or cardiomyopathy.
>
> ◆ While the overall prognosis is guarded, advances in medication, special pacing techniques, and heart transplantation have changed the overall course of cardiac failure.

The term congestive heart failure (CHF) refers to a combination of shortness of breath, fatigue, weakness, and swelling (oedema) of the legs due to ineffective pumping by the heart. Most cases of cardiac failure are due to a weakened heart muscle as a result of a large infarction, cardiac muscle disease (cardiomyopathy), or untreated hypertension. However, in more than 30% of cases, heart contractility is normal or near-normal and the main problem is stiffening of the heart muscle, so that the ventricular filling is impaired. This special type of heart failure has been increasingly recognized over the last 30 years and is more prevalent in women and the elderly, especially in the presence of diabetes or hypertension.

Finally, valvular heart disease or some rhythm disturbances may be responsible for CHF symptoms, although the ventricular contractility is normal. Also, many non-cardiac conditions may mimic congestive heart failure and, conversely, patients with severely diseased hearts may be only mildly symptomatic. Therefore, in newly diagnosed patients without a previous cardiac history, cardiac failure is a clinical diagnosis that should be regarded as a 'first-line' assessment and working hypothesis only, which has to be completed by further investigations to confirm the diagnosis and identify the actual mechanism.

Symptoms of cardiac failure

Cardiac failure should not be confused with evidence of decreased pumping function of the heart obtained from various cardiac tests. In these cases we may diagnose ventricular dysfunction, but the term heart failure is used when symptoms develop. A functional scale is frequently used to grade symptom severity and monitor response to treatment or need for further action (Table 8.1).

Table 8.1 New York Association functional classification heart failure symptoms

Functional class	Symptom occurrence
I	Only with intense above-average effort
II	With moderate effort
III	With minimal effort
IV	At rest

Suggestive heart failure symptoms are described below.

Shortness of breath

This is a very common complaint which can also occur in non-cardiac conditions, such as lung diseases and obesity, and the differential diagnosis may be challenging. The following features are strongly suggestive of heart failure.

◆ Worsening with exercise and improvement at rest.

◆ Clear worsening with lying down (orthopnoea), prompting the patient instinctively to use more pillows to avoid lying flat. In fact, 'How many pillows do you use?' is a frequent question that is asked when heart failure is suspected. In more severe cases, the patients report waking up suddenly at night and having to assume a seating position to be relieved (paroxysmal nocturnal dyspnoea). Breathing difficulties that are not worsened by lying down are unlikely to be cardiac in origin.

Fatigue

Patients with advanced heart failure frequently report general fatigue and 'lack of energy'. Again, this is a very non-specific complaint, found in other conditions as well, and should not be used on its own to make a diagnosis

Cough

Generally, coughing is associated more with lung conditions, but it may also accompany heart failure. Not infrequently, patients with recent onset of CHF are treated for suspected chest infections. The following should raise suspicion that a persistent cough could be due to heart failure:

◆ recent onset of coughing with mucus-tinged or slightly blood-tinged sputum, without any other evidence of chest infection, especially if associated with other signs of heart failure

◆ cough exacerbated by lying flat.

Leg oedema (swelling)

Patients with advanced heart failure tend to retain water and this may become apparent as swelling of the legs. In fact, many presumptive diagnoses of CHF are made because of leg oedema. However, leg oedema may also be related to other conditions, such as diseases of the veins, obesity, or the use of some common drugs such as amlodipine. Oedema involving one leg preferentially or as an isolated finding is unlikely to be cardiac in origin.

Tests to confirm and further evaluate patients with suspected heart failure

For any practical purpose, echocardiography is today a mandatory test in the evaluation of patients with heart failure. After an echocardiographic scan, it should be possible to answer the following questions.

- Are there findings that can confirm and explain the diagnosis of heart failure?
- Is the case suitable for medical treatment only or could there be a benefit from surgical or special pacing techniques as well?
- Is there a need for further investigations?

Frequently, based on your clinical history, symptoms, and chest X-ray findings, your doctor may decide that the diagnosis is likely enough to start specific heart failure treatment, but still expect to be scheduled for an echo scan for further evaluation. Once the diagnosis of heart failure is established, depending on the specifics of your case, you may undergo a special form of exercise test to assess your symptoms objectively and an angiogram to advance the diagnosis further.

Heart failure treatment

Until the late 1960s, heart failure treatment consisted only of diuretics and digoxin. These were variably effective in controlling symptoms, but had no effect on the overall course and prognosis of the disease, and the mortality was very high, with less than 50% of patients expected to remain alive for more than a few years once severe symptoms developed.

Currently, heart failure treatment includes medications and technologies targeting not only symptoms, but also disease progression and prognosis. Together with more widespread use of revascularization techniques, increased hospitalization rates in specialist services, and supportive community heart failure networks, this multipronged approach is responsible for better symptom control and a reported decrease in heart failure mortality.

Drug treatment of heart failure (see also Chapter 14)

Today, the standard treatment of a patient with heart failure is expected to include the following.

- Diuretics: given to promote diuresis and unload the body of excess fluids, and thus relieve symptoms such as shortness of breath and leg swelling.
- Beta-blockers: prescribed in most cases of heart failure due to decreased ventricular contractility. They have been shown both to alleviate symptoms and to improve survival.

- ACE inhibitors: a cornerstone of CHF treatment, ACE inhibitors lessen symptoms, decrease mortality, and may prevent further enlargement and weakening of the heart.

- Digoxin: less used currently in the treatment of heart failure, digoxin is still considered in the presence of atrial fibrillation or if symptoms persist despite appropriate treatment.

Non-drug-based treatment of heart failure

Biventricular pacing (see also Chapter 15)

Numerous patients who remain symptomatic despite conventional treatment may benefit from implantation of special pacemakers (biventricular pacemakers) that improve the contractility of the ventricle by ensuring that all its segments contract synchronously.

Left ventricular assist devices (LVAD)

These are sophisticated pumping devices which are surgically inserted and connected to the heart to work in parallel with it and support its pumping action. LVADs are not a long-term solution but rather a bridging procedure in candidates for heart transplantation whose heart failure is so severe that their short-term survival is very poor.

Heart transplant

Heart transplantation, pioneered by Christian Barnard in 1967 in South Africa, may be the only option for patients with severely diseased ventricles and severe heart failure despite optimal treatment. Heart failure symptoms resolve and long-term survival is dramatically improved, but these patients are put on chronic immunosuppressive treatment and are under continuous monitoring to detect rejection of the new heart which, together with infection and accelerated coronary disease, is the main problem after transplant. Heart transplantation procedures are relatively limited to patients who are otherwise free from any disease that may limit their survival. A stable psychological profile is also important, as life after heart transplant is not easy and involves a lot of self-discipline and readiness to submit to a strict medication regime and follow-up schedule. Even for those deemed suitable, the odds of having the procedure are limited by the lack of donors. Currently, about one-third of the patients on the heart transplantation list in the UK receive a heart transplant.

9
Congenital heart diseases

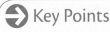 **Key Points**

♦ Congenital heart diseases (CHDs) are a group of cardiac malformations that patients are born with.

♦ Simple instances of CHD can easily be corrected and have an excellent prognosis.

♦ The most frequently encountered forms of CHD are atrial and ventricular septal defects and bicuspid aortic valve.

♦ The majority of patients with simple CHDs which have been successfully corrected have a normal life expectancy and quality of life.

Congenital heart defects affect up to 1% of all live births. Although many cases of CHD occur without an identifiable cause, some conditions are associated with an increased risk of being born with a cardiac malformation:

♦ family history of CHD or complex genetic disorders, such as Down syndrome

♦ viral infection during pregnancy, such as rubella (German measles)

♦ diabetes

♦ use of alcohol and recreational drugs

♦ use of certain medications, such as some anti-epileptic, antidepressive, or anticoagulant drugs, especially during the first trimester of pregnancy.

The formation of the organs is completed by the end of the third month of pregnancy, so this first trimester is the most vulnerable in terms of exposure to drugs, irradiation, or infections. If you are pregnant, you should consult your doctor or pharmacist before using any medication.

Some congenital heart diseases may be considered simple (atrial or ventricular septal defect, patent ductus arteriosus), while others are complex with more than one malformation (tetralogy of Fallot) or with major distortions of the cardiac anatomy. Some CHDs are obvious at birth or in early childhood, being associated with heart failure, failure to thrive, or repeated pulmonary infections, and require early or emergency correction, others are diagnosed only in adult life because of complications, and others may be totally asymptomatic and devoid of complications and found incidentally. The overall prognosis for CHD has improved dramatically, with more than three-quarters of children expected to reach adulthood, and good odds for a normal life and survival rates of almost 100% for those with simple forms of CHD. Owing to the scope of this book, only the the most frequent and uncomplicated forms of CHD that are encountered during adult life are described here.

Atrial septal defect (ASD)

Normally, the two atria are separated by an inter-atrial wall (septum). ASD, which is encountered in about 7% of CHD cases, is a condition where there is communication between the left and right atria. As a result, some blood is shunted from the left atrium to the right atrium because of differences in pressure.

Patients with small ASDs are asymptomatic, do not need any special treatment or activity limitations, and are eventually diagnosed during an echocardiographic study. In addition, unlike patients with other forms of CHD they are not at risk of infectious endocarditis.

Patients with larger ASDs are diagnosed either during childhood or later through typical findings on cardiac examinations. They tend to be asymptomatic until they reach their fourth decade, when they may complain of fatigue and shortness of breath, and have rhythm disturbances.

Most cases of large ASDs do need surgery in order to prevent progressive enlargement of the right heart cavities and possible damage to the lungs cuased by the increased blood flow. This operation is considered quite simple, and transvenous catheter-based techniques for ASD closure without open-heart surgery have recently become available.

Patent foramen ovale (PFO)

Unlike ASD, where there is a real defect in the inter-atrial septum, in PFO the septum is well built but its components are not well positioned one against the other. This results in a valve-like opening which allows blood to be shunted from the right to the left atrium. Patent foramen ovale (Latin: oval hole) is the persistence in adult life of a communication that normally exists in the fetal heart but closes at birth. It is quite a frequent finding, and is described in up to 25% of the general population.

There are no symptoms or haemodynamic abnormalities related to a PFO, and the vast majority of those affected tolerate this condition very well and in fact are not aware of it. Of late, a possible association between migraine and PFO has been described, possibly because of passage of some metabolites directly into the circulation without being filtered by the lungs. Also, some cases of stroke, especially in young individuals, may be related to passage into the circulation of small clots that would normally have been trapped by the lungs. When this relationship is established, the PFO may be closed using a catheter technique, as for ASD, although the indications and best strategies for this procedure are still under evaluation. The diagnosis of PFO is easily made with echocardiography.

Ventricular septal defect (VSD)

In these patients there is a defect in the interventricular septum which allows communication between the ventricles, with resulting shunting of blood from the left to the right ventricle. Isolated VSD is the second most frequent congenital heart disease after bicuspid aortic valve, representing about 20% of CHD cases. Many small VSDs close spontaneously in childhood. Patients with small VSDs have impressive murmurs on physical examination, but are otherwise asymptomatic, lead a perfectly normal life, and do not need surgery or any other treatment. Large VSDs may progress to heart failure or pulmonary complications and therefore do need surgery, as do large ASDs.

Bicuspid aortic valve (BAV)

The aortic valve normally consists of three cusps. In about 1% of individuals a two-cusp aortic valve is found; this is the most frequent form of CHD. During childhood and young to middle age, there is no disturbance related to the valve, the affected individuals are asymptomatic, and the anomaly is suspected during a routine examination due to a specific murmur and confirmed by echocardiography, at which time any possibly associated abnormalities are detected. Young patients with isolated BAV found incidentally need no treatment or activity limitations, but the diagnosis should be documented in their medical records to ensure follow-up. Since the condition may be familial, screening of first-degree relatives is recommended. With advancing age, about a third of these valves become narrowed (stenotic) and/or leaky (regurgitant, incompetent) and may need surgery.

Pulmonary stenosis (PS)

This is another frequent congenital heart disease, representing about 10% of all cases of CHD. In these patients, the pulmonary valve is deformed and stenotic, making it more difficult for the right ventricle to pump blood into the pulmonary artery. PS is frequently diagnosed by chance when a cardiac murmur is detected. Most cases are mild and asymptomatic and do not progress, so there is no need for treatment and there are no functional limitations in affected individuals. More severe cases are generally resolved during childhood with either a balloon valvuloplasty or surgery.

Patent ductus arteriosus (PDA)

The ductus arteriosus (Latin: arterial channel) is a vascular conduit connecting the pulmonary artery to the aorta. In the foetus it allows shunting of oxygenated blood directly to the aorta, thus avoiding the fetal lungs, which are not functional. Immediately after birth, the fetal circulation pattern is replaced by the adult pattern, and the lungs are fully included in the circulation to allow blood oxygenation and the ductus slowly constricts until it closes completely. Failure of this process and persistence of this communication beyond a few months after birth is called patent ductus arteriosus and is a frequent (5–10%) form of CHD. Large PDAs may present with various degrees of heart failure. Most cases of haemodynamically significant PDAs are discovered and closed during childhood. Small PDAs may remain completely asymptomatic and be incidentally discovered in adult life because of a typical cardiac murmur. Owing to a theoretical risk of infection at the site, even small PDAs are generally electively closed either surgically or using a catheter-based procedure in which a specially designed coil is placed in the conduit, leading to its obliteration.

 Frequently Asked Questions

Q: My 8-year-old son has been seen by our GP because of a cold. He told us that he heard a murmur over his heart and an echocardiography should be done to rule out a problem. We are worried now. Is this something serious?

A: Most probably not. Murmurs are sounds made by the blood flowing through the heart. They do not necessarily mean that disease is present and they are quite common, especially in children and young individuals who have a more dynamic blood flow. As a rule, a mild murmur accidentally heard in an otherwise healthy individual is most probably of no consequence. Whether to refer the patient for cardiological work-up or not should be your GP's decision.

Q: My 13-year-old daughter is a perfectly healthy and happy teenager. When she was born, we were told that she had a small 'hole' in her heart but there was no need to worry and no treatment was necessary. However, now that she has grown and is very active physically, we are worried about her heart condition. Is it possible to have a 'hole' in the heart and yet be a normal healthy person?

A: The answer is 'yes'. Obviously you have to discuss this in detail with your cardiologist and some follow-up may be necessary, but there are cases of small openings in the walls that separate the cardiac chambers that have no impact at all and do not need treatment. Some of them even close spontaneously with age. To simplify things, they are sometimes referred to as 'small holes' in the heart when talking to the child's parents.

10

Cardiomyopathies and arrhythmogenic syndromes

 Key Points

- The cardiac muscle is primarily involved in cardiomyopathies(CMPs).
- The most frequent CMPs encountered in clinical practice are a dilated form, associated with decreased ventricular contractility, and a hypertrophic form, where the heart muscle is abnormally thick.
- CMPs may be associated with severe heart failure and life-threatening arrhythmias.
- Fatal arrhythmias are possible in young individuals with organically normal hearts but rare genetic conditions: channelopathies.
- Family screening is indicated in healthy relatives of affected individuals.

In cardiomyopathies there is a primary injury of the cardiac muscle itself, not related to hypertension or significant coronary or valvular disease. In some cases a specific responsible agent or a background disease can be identified:

- genetic defects
- some neurological and metabolic conditions
- alcohol overuse
- toxins
- infections
- lack of specific nutrients.

Our understanding of these diseases is evolving, leading to changes in classification criteria and continuous revision of the boundaries between primary and secondary cases. Echocardiography plays a central role in the assessment of cardiomyopathies, together with magnetic resonance and genetic tests. The most frequently encountered cardiomyopathies are described below.

Dilated cardiomyopathy (DCMP)

In these patients the heart progressively dilates and its contractile force diminishes until the patient develops congestive heart failure and may be at risk for life-threatening arrhythmias.

Idiopathic CMP

When no aetiology is found, DCMP is considered to be idiopathic. The actual frequency of idiopathic DCMP in the general population is not known. Some cases are believed to follow a previous viral infection and some probably have a genetic component, since in a quarter of these patients there is evidence of familial involvement as well. Echo and ECG screening is recommended for first-degree relatives.

Peripartum cardiomyopathy (PPCMP)

PPCMP is a rare form of DCMP with onset during the last month of pregnancy or within a few months after delivery. The cause of PPCMP is not clear, but it is more frequent in women over 30 years of age and in pregnancies complicated by hypertension. Recovery is expected in about 50% of cases, but there are recurrences in subsequent pregnancies in up to 40%. Therefore new pregnancies are best avoided, especially in the absence of full recovery after the first episode.

Alcohol-induced DCMP

Prolonged and excessive use of alcohol is a relatively frequent cause of DCMP. In some cases, the damage is reversible once alcohol consumption stops.

DCMP management

Patients with newly diagnosed DCMP should be assessed for treatable causes and for risk stratification. The treatment is the standard treatment for congestive heart failure. Implantable defibrillators, biventricular pacing, or heart transplantation are considered in suitable cases.

Hypertrophic cardiomyopathy (HCM)

HCM was first described in the late 1950s. These patients have an abnormally thick (hypertrophic) heart muscle in the absence of hypertension or valvular heart disease. The reason is a genetic anomaly which induces an abnormal disorganized structure of the heart muscle. HCMP is thought to be present in about one in 500 of the general population. Most cases are familial, with each child of an affected person having a 50% chance of having the condition, irrespective of gender. The clinical expression may be very mild, and so the disease may not be recognized unless specifically sought. In typical cases, there is severe thickening of the ventricular, walls, mainly of the interventricular septum, with a striking echocardiographic appearance. The abnormal myocardial structure and the thick ventricular walls are responsible for the main consequences of the disease.

◆ A 'stiff' heart, responsible for a slow filling of the ventricle, resulting in symptoms of heart failure.

◆ A tendency for both ventricular and supraventricular arrhythmias, some of them life threatening.

◆ An abnormal motion of the mitral valve, which moves towards the septum and impedes the emptying of the ventricle in systole (obstructive HCM), noted in about a quarter of patients.

HCM may become apparent at any age, but typically it is recognized after puberty or in the twenties. Patients may be asymptomatic and the disease is eventually diagnosed by echocardiography, following the finding of a cardiac murmur or an abnormal ECG.

Symptomatic individuals suffer from:

◆ shortness of breath

◆ chest pain

◆ fatigue

◆ palpitations.

There is a risk of sudden death, especially in young patients or those with relatives who died suddenly, and HCM is the most common cause of sudden death in the young individuals. The treatment includes beta-blockers and/or calcium-channel blockers, and anti-arrhythmic drugs. In selected severe cases of obstructive CMP, surgical resection of part of the thickened septum can relieve most of the symptoms. Recently, a non-surgical alternative has been suggested in which alcohol is injected into a branch of the coronary artery so that part of the thickened cardiac muscle is destroyed. Defibrillators are used in patients judged at risk of sudden death.

Athlete's heart

Athletes engaged in prolonged and strenuous training, generally at competition level, may present with adaptive cardiac changes resulting in an ECG and echocardiographic picture similar to that of HCMP, although the degree of hypertrophy is less marked. This condition, known as 'athlete's heart' may raise difficult issues of differential diagnosis, because individuals with true HCMP should not participate in intense sportive activities. Various criteria are available to differentiate between the two entities. Occasionally, regression of left ventricular hypertrophy after ceasing training helps with the final diagnosis.

Arrhythmogenic right ventricular cardiomyopathy (ARVC)

ARVC, first described in France in the late 1970s, is an uncommon condition, also genetically determined, which leads to degenerative and fatty infiltrative changes in the right ventricle. Affected individuals may develop signs of right heart failure (leg swelling, fatigue), but the main concern is of life-threatening ventricular arrhythmias. ARVC, together with HCMP, is the most common cause of sudden death in the young. Once the condition is suspected, because of symptoms and ECG evidence of arrhythmias originating in the right ventricle or a positive family history, the diagnosis is confirmed by echocardiography and MR scanning. These patients will receive standard treatment for heart failure, when needed. The best way to prevent sudden death is implantation of a defibrillator.

Arrhythmogenic syndromes

In addition to the cardiomyopathies described above, there exists a group of rare diseases, also genetically determined, which have in common a tendency for life-threatening arrhythmias despite the lack of identifiable organic heart pathology. Since they are related to abnormalities of sodium, potassium, or calcium ion channels at myocardial cell level, they are collectively known as channelopathies. They are responsible for some otherwise unexplained instances of arrhythmic sudden death. The most common channelopathies are long QT syndrome (LQTS) and Brugada syndrome. Both may present with palpitations or syncope and evidence of ventricular arrhythmia.

The diagnosis may be suggested by a positive family history and typical ECG appearance, but this is not always obvious and a high degree of suspicion may be necessary. High-risk cases are referred for implantable defibrillators, but as a rule the investigation and management of these rare disorders should be the responsibility of experts who specialize in inherited arrhythmogenic conditions.

Family screening in patients with cardiomyopathies and arrhythmogenic syndromes

Most of the conditions described in this chapter are genetically determined and frequently run in families. Since sudden death can be the first manifestation of the disease, the importance of early detection in asymptomatic individuals cannot be overemphasized. Ideally, a genetic test should be able to identify the defect in patient's relatives. However, this is not always practical and reliable for the following reasons.

◆ Lack of sufficient knowledge about all possible genes involved in one disease and low sensitivity of available tests (genetical tests are negative in 30–50% of patients with HCMP and in an even higher proportion in other conditions).

◆ High costs and limited availability of genetic testing.

◆ Lack of certainty about the meaning of a positive test in an asymptomatic relative: not all the carriers of the abnormal gene develop the disease, and some may develop a mild form of it.

As things stand now, genetic testing may be considered in selected cases but is not used routinely.

Clinical screening

Full clinical and echocardiographic screening is recommended in asymptomatic first-degree relatives (parents, siblings, children) of patients with manifest cardiomyopathies or channelopathies. A negative result does not necessarily mean that the disease is not present, since the clinical onset may be delayed and various conditions behave differently.

In HCMP, the clinical picture may become apparent during the pubertal growth spurt and is unlikely to occur after growth is completed. Therefore children from families with HCMP are followed up with ECG and echocardiography until their twenties.

ARVC may develop later in life. Therefore repeated follow-up is recommended without clear age limits.

11

Pericarditis and myocarditis

 Key Points

- These conditions refer to an inflammation of the pericardium (the envelope of the heart) or the cardiac muscle.

- The cause is generally thought to be a viral infection, although frequently this cannot be proved. Alternatively, they may be related to a non-cardiac disease or to certain drugs.

- The two conditions may coexist or they may develop as separate entities.

Pericarditis

The clinical picture ranges from a flu-like syndrome with chest discomfort to excruciating chest pain with ECG changes and evidence of pericardial fluid. The pain is typically sharp and worsened by breathing, coughing, or movements, and thus is easily differentiated from anginal pain. Most cases are benign and self-limiting, and require only rest and anti-inflammatory medication. Rare cases have a protracted recurrent course and may need prolonged treatment.

Myocarditis

The typical presentation of myocarditis is of acute onset of otherwise unexplained heart failure. The ECG may show non-specific changes, but the diagnosis rests on echocardiography which will show decreased ventricular contractility, generally with a diffuse distribution, unlike coronary disease, although the differential diagnosis may be difficult. A history of a recent viral-like disease (fever, diarrhoea, muscular pains) may be present occasionally but this is not always the case. Most cases are self-limiting and have a good prognosis. The treatment in the acute phase is standard heart failure treatment which can gradually be stopped when the condition improves. Rare cases result in extreme life-threatening heart failure requiring intensive care treatment, use of ventricular assist devices, and possibly heart transplantation. Some cases of idiopathic dilated cardiomyopathy are thought to represent the final stage of slowly evolving myocarditis which was previously unrecognized.

12
Valvular heart disease

Key Points

- Any of the four cardiac valves (see Chapter 1, Figure 1.3) can be diseased, but the mitral and aortic valves are mainly affected.

- The valves can be either narrowed with limited opening (stenotic) or with incomplete closure (incompetent or regurgitant). A combination of both lesions is also possible and more than one valve can be affected.

- Rheumatic heart disease used to the main aetiology of valvular heart disease (VHD), but over the last 50 years its prevalence decreased in the developed countries and, except for mitral stenosis, most cases of valvular disease are now related to degenerative or age-related mechanisms.

- Echocardiography is the best method available for assessing VHD.

- Slowly developing valve lesions are well tolerated until the advanced stages.

- Once symptoms occur the valve has to be replaced or repaired. Either mechanical or tissue (biological) valves can be used.

Mitral stenosis (MS)

In these patients, mainly women, the mitral valve does not fully open and so there is restriction to blood flow from the left atrium to the left ventricle. The disease is secondary to rheumatic fever, which is a possible complication of a streptococcal infection manifesting itself as a sore throat in childhood. Improved hygiene and prompt antibiotic treatment of sore throats brought in a dramatic decrease in the frequency of the disease in the Western world after the Second World War, although it is still a problem in developing countries. Affected individuals can be mildly symptomatic, or they can increasingly complain of shortness of breath and palpitations and develop heart failure and atrial fibrillation. MS patients with atrial fibrillation are at high risk of stroke and have a strong indication for anticoagulation. Mild disease can be managed conservatively, but in severe symptomatic cases the mitral valve has to be replaced. In selected patients the mitral valve can be opened using a special balloon-tipped catheter and thus surgery is avoided. Untreated cases may evolve to severe heart failure, but overall prognosis is excellent with appropriate management.

Mitral regurgitation (MR)

With MR, the mitral valve fails to close fully, allowing the blood to flow back from the ventricle into the atrium during systole. The backward build of pressure in the lungs and the need for the ventricle to cope with increased amounts of blood and maintain a normal cardiac output are responsible for the symptoms of shortness of breath and gradual enlargement and weakening of the heart. MR used to be mainly a result of rheumatic disease, but currently most cases are due to degenerative changes or coronary heart disease. Mild and moderate cases are generally very well tolerated for long periods of time and do not need specific treatment, although monitoring may be indicated to detect possible progression. Even severe cases can also be well tolerated for a long period, but they will generally need either valve replacement or surgical repair at some point. Main symptoms are shortness of breath and fatigue, evolving to frank heart failure in neglected cases. Ideally, surgery should be performed when minimal symptoms develop and before there is a\ceny damage to the left ventricle.

Mitral valve prolapse (MVP)

In the general population, about 2–3% of individuals present with variable degrees of thickening of the mitral valve, which also has an abnormal bowing (prolapse) of one or both leaflets into the left atrium in systole. Initially, this condition, which is due to degenerative changes in the mitral valve structure, was associated with a large array of possible symptoms and complications, ranging from chest pain to arrhythmias and stroke. However, recent data suggest a much lower rate of complications and an overall benign course in the majority of cases. Nevertheless, the degenerative changes in the mitral valve can progress until the valve becomes incompetent. In the Western world, MVP currently represents the most frequent reason for surgical intervention for severe mitral regurgitation.

Aortic stenosis (AS)

In these patients the aortic valve does not open freely, and so high pressure has to be generated by the left ventricle to pump the blood in the aorta. Initially, the ventricle thickens and is able to cope with the burden for long periods of time, but eventually it starts to fail and a heart failure picture may develop. AS is currently the most frequent valvular heart disease. It is due to progressive thickening and calcification of the valve, and its prevalence increases in the elderly population. The mechanism responsible for AS seems to be, at least at the beginning, an inflammatory process, very much like vascular atherosclerotic changes, followed by leaflet thickening. Abnormal blood flow through the valve may promote and accelerate these changes, and indeed about half of patients with AS have a bicuspid aortic valve. Cases of congenital aortic stenosis are detected in childhood and rheumatic AS is rare today. The diagnosis is suggested by a typical harsh murmur and is confirmed by echocardiography. When symptomatic, AS manifests itself with:

◆ shortness of breath, mainly exertional and other features of heart failure

◆ angina-like chest pain, which can occur even in the absence of coronary disease

◆ dizziness or frank syncope, reflecting a critical reduction in cardiac output.

Once these symptoms have developed, or if there is echocardiographic evidence of decrease in left ventricular contractility, there is a clear indication for aortic valve replacement. Non-surgical catheter-based valve-replacement techniques have recently become available for cases of high surgical risk.

Aortic regurgitation (AR)

If the aortic valve fails to close fully during diastole, blood flows back from the aorta into the ventricle. As a result, the left ventricle progressively enlarges to accommodate the increased amount of blood, and eventually its contractility decreases. Aortic regurgitation occurs mainly because of an inborn defect, such as a bicuspid aortic valve, or when the valve orifice is stretched by disease, resulting in a progressive enlargement of the aortic root. AR is suspected when a typical diastolic murmur is heard or a large heart is noted on chest radiography. Echocardiography provides diagnostic confirmation and clarifies the mechanism responsible. Like other valve disease, AR is well tolerated for a long time. Once heart failure symptoms develop or the left ventricle enlarges beyond critical dimensions, valve replacement is necessary.

Surgery for valvular heart disease

Valve-replacement surgery started in the early 1950s. Today valve surgery is a highly sophisticated procedure which can be performed as either valve replacement or valve repair. Catheter-based and minimally invasive procedures are also continuously being developed to avoid open-heart surgery in selected cases. Each kind of valvular intervention has its specific advantages and drawbacks, and your surgeon will discuss which one would be the best option in your case. Operative results are very good, and the overall mortality may be less than 5%, depending on the characteristics of the case.

Valve replacement

Valve replacement can be performed using either metallic or biological (generally made from animal valve tissue) prostheses.

Metallic prosthetic valves

The first prosthetic valves consisted of a moving ball contained in a metallic cage. These valves had an excellent record of durability, but were bulky and therefore difficult to use in some cases, and were occasionally noisy enough to be heard by the patient or even those surrounding him. Valve design has evolved continuously, and today's mechanical valves are generally a bi-leaflet 'butterfly-like' type, have a low profile with excellent haemodynamic characteristics, and are silent and well tolerated. The main advantage of prosthetic valves is their almost unlimited durability. However, clot formation may be promoted on their surfaces, with a risk of valve malfunction or stroke. This risk is higher for valves in the mitral position than in the aortic position and in the presence of atrial fibrillation or decreased ventricular contractility. Therefore all patients with mechanical valves need chronic anticoagulation, generally with warfarin, and aspirin may be added as well. The target international normalized ratio (INR) for patients with mechanical valves is in the range 2.5–3.5, i.e. higher than for atrial fibrillation (see Chapter 14). The use of anticoagulation effectively reduces the risk of clot formation to as low as 1% per patient-year, depending on the type of valve, the position, and coexisting cardiac conditions.

Tissue (biological) prosthetic valves

Tissue valves are typically manufactured from a valve explanted from a pig (porcine valves) or from bovine pericardium and mounted on a strut structure, although occasionally they are left un-mounted and implanted as such. Their foremost advantage is that, except for a few months after surgery, they do not require anticoagulation, making them an attractive option when chronic anticoagulation is contraindicated or logistically difficult. The main drawback of biological valves is their relatively short lifetime compared with mechanical valves. The tissue leaflets are expected to deteriorate and a repeat operation may be required after 10–15 years, although individual variations are wide. The lifetime of bioprosthetic valves tends to be shorter in youngsters, presumably because of their more dynamic circulation; therefore they are not generally considered in this age group. An exception to this is women of child-bearing age because warfarin is contraindicated in pregnancy. However, they should be aware that they may need a repeat operation in the future. On the other hand, bioprosthetic valves are a good option in the elderly and are frequently used for patients over the age of 65.

Valvular repair

Incompetent aortic valves in young individuals are occasionally repaired rather than replaced, but most valvular repairs are performed for mitral incompetence. In fact, whenever possible, mitral valve repair is preferred over replacement since it is associated with preservation of ventricular and valvular structures, has a very low operative risk, does not require long-term anticoagulation as mechanical prostheses do, and does not have the durability issues of bioprosthetic valves. The technique involves resecting, replacing, and remodelling the affected leaflet(s), and frequently inserting a ring to ensure good closure of the leaflets. The drawbacks of the method are that it is not suitable for all valve pathologies (severely damaged valves may not be repaired) and, especially for complex repairs, requires a higher level of expertise than valve replacement.

Infective endocarditis

Infection of inner layer of the heart is called infective endocarditis (IE), and it almost always involves the heart valves. The term is also used for prosthetic valves or for non-valvular structures, such as ventricular septal defect. Infection of pacemaker electrodes is called pacemaker endocarditis. Any bacteria can cause endocarditis, but some, such as streptococci and staphylococci, are encountered more frequently.

Why does endocarditis happen?

IE happens when micro-organisms reach the blood flow and infect one or more cardiac valves. The port of entry is occasionally obvious, such as an open wound or a non-sterile intravenous injection. Frequently, however, it cannot be identified, or it is assumed that a procedure, such as a bleeding dental procedure, 'opens the gates' for micro-organisms normally existing within body cavities to reach the blood flow. IE can occur in anyone, but it is most likely to happen in patients with pre-existing valvular problems or intra-cardiac foreign bodies, whose surface can be colonized more easily by bacteria. In fact, aggressive micro-organisms, such as staphylococci, may infect any valve, but less virulent ones will generally only infect valves that are already damaged.

Who is at risk?

Overall, IE is a rare disease in the general population. The following conditions are considered to raise the risk of developing infective endocarditis:

- existing valvular disease
- prosthetic valves
- obstructive hypertrophic cardiomyopathy
- most types of non-corrected congenital heart disease (not simple ASD).

How can IE be prevented?

Until recently, antibiotics were recommended in these patients before dental and some urological or genital procedures, especially if associated with bleeding. However, the relationship between these procedures and subsequent endocarditis, and the practical value of antibiotic prophylaxis have recently been questioned. In the UK, the National Institutes for Clinical Excellence (NICE) no longer recommends antibiotic prophylaxis before dental or urogenital procedures for anyone. American and European guidelines still recommend it, but limit it to patients judged to be at high risk (previous endocarditis, prosthetic valves, complex congenital heart disease).

As general measures, the following are recommended to decrease the risk of endocarditis:

* maintain good oral hygiene
* avoid potential ports of entry for infections such as body piercing
* do not inject illicit substances.

How is endocarditis recognized?

The clinical picture depends very much on the virulence of the micro-organism and the degree of valvular damage. Some patients present with a dramatic picture of acute febrile disease and rapidly evolving heart failure, while others have a prolonged course of intermittent mild fever, sweats, and generally being unwell. Complications, such as stroke or slowly progressive heart failure, may also be the presenting symptom. The diagnosis is based on positive blood cultures and evidence of valvular damage, generally by echocardiography which plays a crucial role in the management of IE. Occasionally, patients with IE have negative blood cultures after recent treatment with antibiotics by their GP for a suspected common infection. This may hinder a quick diagnosis; therefore patients at risk for IE who present with an unclear febrile disease should not be prescribed antibiotics straightforwardly unless the diagnosis is clear.

What are the risks and complications of endocarditis?

Bacterial multiplication and local inflammatory reaction result in specific growths, called vegetations, on the valve leaflets which further damage the valve. In addition, fragments of large vegetations may detach and cause a stroke. Together with the general effects of the infection, severe valvular damage and stroke are the most feared complications of IE.

How is endocarditis treated?

IE is treated with high doses of antibiotics, frequently in combinations of two or three, given intravenously over a long period of time (usually 6 weeks). If there is no response to antibiotics or there is evidence of rapid valve destruction and heart failure, early or even emergency surgery may be necessary. Even some patients who respond well and become asymptomatic may still need valve surgery at a later stage. Overall, most patients respond to treatment, but endocarditis remains a serious disease. The earlier it is recognized and treated, the better is the outcome.

13

Sudden cardiac death

 Key Points

- The majority of sudden cardiac death (SCD) cases are due to an arrhythmia: ventricular tachycardia or fibrillation.
- Most cases of SCD occur in individuals with organic heart disease.
- The most likely cause in young individuals is a cardiomyopathy, while in the elderly it is coronary disease.
- The survival of individuals at risk has been dramatically improved by the use of implantable defibrillators.

SCD is defined as the unexpected occurrence of death in an individual who has been in a stable condition during the previous 24 hours, although some definitions use a 1 hour cut-off. SCD is usually arrhythmic in nature, i.e. it is due to an arrhythmia such as sustained ventricular tachycardia or ventricular fibrillation, although bradyarrhythmias are identified in 20–30% of cases. Most cases of SCD occur in individuals with some form of organic heart disease. The prevention of SCD has made tremendous advances because of the identification of individuals at risk (decreased left ventricular function, cardiomyopathies, arrhythmogenic syndromes, successfully resuscitated patients) and the use of implantable defibrillators.

The challenge is obviously represented by individuals without known heart disease who have their first event. As many as 40% of out-of-hospital cases are unwitnessed. The odds of immediate survival and lack of significant neurological damage in the long run for witnessed cases depend on the presence 'in the field' of individuals trained in basic life support and the speed of the arrival of highly trained ambulance-based teams, able to deliver advanced resuscitation and life support. Some data suggest a possible 20% rate of survival and hospital discharge for patients with out-of hospital SCD, although the numbers vary greatly in various reports. Community training programmes and availability of automatic external defibrillators in public spaces and on commercial flights may improve these results.

SCD in the middle-aged and elderly

Above the 30–40 years age range, the most likely cause of SCD is coronary artery disease, either in the setting of an acute myocardial infarction or on the background of decreased left ventricular contractility. Most survivors of SCD are found to have extensive coronary disease, and the strongest risk factor for SCD is severely decreased left ventricular function. The importance of regular screening in individuals at risk is emphasized by the fact that SCD can be the first manifestation of coronary disease. Other causes of SCD in this age group are dilated cardiomyopathy, again related to severely decreased left ventricular function, and severe aortic stenosis.

SCD in the young

SCD is a rare but devastating occurrence in this age group. Most cases of SCD below the age of 30 are related to one of the cardiomyopathies or arrhythmogenic syndromes described in Chapter 10. Most instances happen during exercise, but occurrence during sleep is possible with Brugada syndrome and some forms of prolonged QT. The key to prevention is identifying patients at risk, so that they are referred for defibrillator implantation.

Section 3

Treatments

14

Cardiovascular drugs

➜ Key Points

◆ This chapter is dedicated to commonly used cardiovascular drugs. Rarely used drugs, with specific indications and mainly for specialist use, are only briefly mentioned. Drugs are presented using their *generic names*, i.e. a simplified pharmacological name, not related to a particular manufacturer.

◆ Various manufacturers provide different *trade names*. Usually, the box/vial and the leaflet with your medication will mention both the generic and the trade names.

◆ Some cardiac drugs, such as nitrates, have a narrow indication (symptomatic relief of angina), while others, such as beta-blockers or angiotensin-converting enzyme (ACE) inhibitors have a wide spectrum of indications. You may have friends with different cardiac conditions, who are treated with the same drugs.

◆ There is practically no medication that is free of potential side effects. The decision whether to use it or not depends on the perceived benefit–risk ratio for a given patient.

◆ Some side effects are only consequences of the expected effects of the drugs which are exaggerated due to the dose used, drug interactions, or increased susceptibility of a given patient, while others represent true side effects which are not related to the primary action of the drug.

◆ Non-specific allergic reactions can occur with any drug. If you notice something unusual after starting a new medication, this can be related to it even if it is not on the list of frequent side effects.

There is no ideal classification of the wide array of medications that a twenty-first century cardiologist may use to treat cardiac patients. Drugs can be described in terms of their chemical structure, mode of action, or main indications, and each of these criteria may be more or less suitable according to the target audience and the main purpose of the presentation.

The approach adopted here is to use the broad categories accepted for drug description in the cardiological literature with emphasis on the following.

- Basic mechanism(s) of action: as necessary to have a good understanding of a given drug.

- Main indication(s): accepted cardiovascular indications (some drugs may also have non-cardiovascular indications).

- Usual dosage and duration of treatment (when appropriate). Occasionally your doctor may prescribe a dose that is significantly lower or higher than the range quoted in this book. This represents his/her clinical decision to use a minimum or a maximum dose in your specific case.

- Specific precautions, contraindications, and typical side effects

A synoptic summary of most common drugs used in cardiovascular medicine is provided in Table 14.1.

Statins

Following research in Japan in the 1970s, statins are currently the most widely used drugs in patients with high cholesterol levels, as they are able to lower cholesterol levels dramatically by 40% or more. They are credited with a significant decrease in cardiovascular risk, and, together with beta-blockers and ACE inhibitors, are among the most valuable additions to the armoury of drugs available to treat cardiac patients. Statins work by inhibiting the HMG-CoA reductase enzyme, which is essential for cholesterol cellular synthesis. As a result, liver cells have less 'own cholesterol' and need to 'capture' more LDL-cholesterol, which is thus cleared from the blood. The main effect of statins is to decrease total and LDL-cholesterol levels, although a modest reduction in triglycerides is also noted. As well as lowering cholesterol, statins are credited with improving the function of vessel walls and with some anti-inflammatory effects. Because of their multiple complex effects, statins are also considered for a variety of non-cardiac conditions such as prevention of fractures in patients with osteoporosis, prevention of Alzheimer's disease, worsening heart failure, and sepsis. However, these indications are only investigational at the moment.

Indications

The indications for statins use are continuously reviewed, and this topic is dealt with in detail in Chapter 4. Briefly, established indications for statins in individuals with cholesterol levels above treatment targets (total cholesterol, 4–5 mmol/litre; LDL-cholesterol, 2–3 mmol/litre) are as follows.

- Secondary prevention: individuals with established atherosclerotic cardiovascular disease (coronary artery disease, ischaemic stroke, aortic aneurysm, peripheral vascular disease).

Table 14.1 Main categories of cardiovascular drugs (note that some of are included in a number of categories because of their wide range of indications

Lipid-lowering drugs	Antiplatelet	Anticoagulants	Anti-anginal/anti-ischaemic drugs	Anti-hypertensive drugs	Cardiac failure drugs	Anti-arrhythmics
Statins	Aspirin	Warfarin	Nitrates	Diuretics	Diuretics	Beta-blockers
Fibrates	Clopidogrel	Heparin	Nicorandil	Beta-blockers	Digoxin	Flecainide
	Dipyridamole		'Pure' heart-rate lowering agents	Alpha-blockers	Beta-blockers	Propafenone
			Beta-blockers	ACE inhibitors/ARBs	ACE inhibitors/ARBs	Sotalol
			Calcium-channel blockers	Central acting agents		Amiodarone

ACE, angiotensin-converting enzyme; ARB, angiotensin receptor blocker.

- Primary prevention: individuals without clinical evidence of atherosclerotic cardiovascular disease but with
  - 10-year calculated risk of cardiovascular disease > 20%
  - diabetes
  - ratio of total cholesterol to HDL-cholesterol greater than 6.

Usual dosage

Several statins are currently on the market. They are very similar, though they may differ slightly in terms of incidence of side effects. As for ACE inhibitors, some of them have more evidence of benefit than others.

- pravastatin: 10–40 mg once daily
- simvastatin: 10–80 mg once daily
- atorvastatin: 10–80 mg once daily.

Statins should be taken in the evening since the HMG-CoA reductase enzyme is at its highest activity level at this time. Consumption of grapefruit juice should be avoided.

Side effects, contraindications, and precautions

Generally, statins are well tolerated. Recognized side effects include the following.

Muscle inflammation and damage (statin myopathy)

A small percentage (5–10%) of patients may develop muscular aches and tenderness. In most cases, this can be solved by using a smaller dose or switching to a different statin. More severe symptoms or a significant rise in creatine kinase (a muscular enzyme) are rare but may dictate cessation of treatment. Significant damage to muscles, resulting in severe complications, is extremely rare. Advanced age, small body size, renal failure, untreated hypothyroidism, and association with a fibrate may predispose to this complication.

Liver damage

Altered liver tests are noted in a minority of patients. Mild changes require monitoring only. Statins should not be given to patients with active liver disease, and caution is advised in those with a history of liver disease or at risk due to alcoholism. Liver function tests should be obtained before starting the treatment and periodically rechecked thereafter.

Digestive intolerance

This is s rarely reported in patients taking statins.

Memory loss

Sporadic reports and discussions in patients' forums mention possible memory loss related to the use of statins. As things stand now, there are no controlled data and no rigorous evidence of a possible deleterious effect of statins on memory. Therefore these concerns are regarded as anecdotal evidence only, counterbalanced by the clear large-scale benefit and positive impact of statins in patients with or at risk of cardiovascular diseases.

Fibrates

Lowering LDL-cholesterol is the main objective when treating patients with or at risk of cardiovascular disease. Triglyceride lowering (see Chapter 4) may be an objective in itself in some genetic conditions with severe hypertriglyc-eridaemia or in cardiac patients, mainly overweight or diabetic, when LDL-cholesterol levels are close to target range but triglycerides are very high despite diet, weight reduction, and exercise. Fibrates (bezafibrate, fenofibrate) are a group of agents which have a more modest effect on LDL-cholesterol but are more effective than statins in lowering triglycerides and increasing the 'good' HDL-cholesterol. They share with statins the risk of myopathy, especially in patients with renal failure. This is of concern, especially when fibrates are used together with statins. This combination is acceptable, but caution should be exercised and generally should be prescribed under specialist control.

Other agents used in the treatment of hyperlipidaemias

Other agents can occasionally be used to control lipid levels, especially when the required dose of statins is not tolerated. Compared with statins, there are fewer data available on their long-term beneficial effects.

- ◆ **Resins** (colestyramine, colestipol) reduce the reabsorption of bile acids, thus depleting the 'cholesterol pool' of the body. These agents were the mainstay of cholesterol-lowering treatment before the advent of statins, but their use was hampered by poor gastric tolerance. They have been largely replaced by ezetimibe (see below).

- ◆ **Ezetimibe** blocks the intestinal absorption of cholesterol. It is used as a supplement to statins when high doses are not effective or not tolerated. Possible diarrhoea and liver impairment have been reported.

- ◆ **Nicotinic acid** is a vitamin B compound that is effective in lowering both LDL-cholesterol and triglycerides and increasing HDL-cholesterol levels. Its use has been limited by side effects, especially flushing, but new products are better tolerated.

Antiplatelet drugs

Platelets (thrombocytes) are normal blood cells involved in the process of stopping bleeding (haemosthasis) and repairing injuries to blood vessels walls. When necessary, they clump together to form a blood clot (thrombus). However, an inappropriate response can occur and initiate the development of a clot that can occlude a coronary artery or a stent, inducing a heart attack or worsening angina. Antiplatelet drugs are used alone or in combination to decrease the odds of abnormal platelet activation. As expected, a slightly increased tendency to bleed is possible, but, except for the very elderly, the odds of major bleeding are low. It is accepted that, despite the slight increase in the risk of bleeding complications, when properly indicated the benefits of antiplatelet agents in preventing cardiovascular events far outweigh their risks.

Aspirin

The chemical compound acetyl salicylic acid is universally known as aspirin, the name under which it was first produced and marketed by the Bayer Company in 1900. In high doses (1–3 g/day), aspirin is used as a pain killer to lower fever and to treat various inflammatory conditions. In much smaller doses (75–150 mg/day), aspirin is used in cardiovascular medicine because of its antiplatelet properties.

Indications

- Primary prevention in patients with increased risk of coronary disease:
    - expected 15% reduction in cardiovascular events.
- Secondary prevention in patients with already established coronary or other atherosclerotic vascular disease:
    - expected 25% reduction in cardiovascular events.
- After CABG or a balloon or stent procedure to open an obstructed artery.
- Secondary prevention of patients after an ischaemic stroke.
- Stroke prevention in low to moderate risk cases of atrial fibrillation.
- In addition to warfarin for selected patients with prosthetic mechanical valves.

In the absence of contraindications, aspirin is given for life in all these cases, except for atrial fibrillation where it can be stopped in selected cases when the arrhythmia has been effectively treated.

Usual dosage

- 75 mg/day (a 300 mg loading dose may be used in acute conditions).

Side effects, contraindications, and precautions

Aspirin at this small dose is generally very well tolerated, although some patients will report some gastric discomfort. In these cases your doctor may either add an antacid or switch you to clopidogrel. There is no need to prescribe an antacid automatically for all patients taking aspirin. There is a small risk of major gastric bleeding, so aspirin should not be prescribed to patients with known peptic disease and/or previous gastric bleeding for whom clopidogrel is generally safer, although not foolproof. There is also a small risk of intracranial bleeding, especially in the elderly or with poorly controlled hypertension.

Some patients, especially the elderly, may report an increased tendency for minor bleeding or easy bruising. Finally, aspirin may be poorly tolerated in a minority of asthmatic patients.

Clopidogrel

Clopidogrel inhibits platelet activity by a mechanism different from that of aspirin. It is used either as an alternative to aspirin for patients with aspirin intolerance or in combination with it when a strong antiplatelet effect is necessary. The aspirin–clopidogrel combination is of proven value following some acute conditions or coronary interventions, but, as expected, the bleeding risks are also increased and so it is generally used for limited periods.

Indications

* As an alternative to aspirin in patients with intolerance or contraindications to aspirin.
* In combination with aspirin:
  * after an acute coronary syndrome: up to 12 months
  * after a coronary intervention with stent implantation: up to 12 months (depending on the type of stent used).

Usual dosage

* 75 mg/day (higher doses are used in acute conditions or before interventions).

Side effects, contraindications, and precautions

Clopidogrel shares with aspirin the risk of increased bleeding but has a better gastric tolerance. Flu-like symptoms have been reported in some patients, but, as for aspirin, the overall tolerance is excellent.

Dipyridamole

Dipyridamole is an antiplatelet agent which also has vasodilator properties. It is generally used in combination with aspirin in patients after an ischaemic stroke. Given intravenously, it is used in some diagnostic tests for coronary disease.

Indications

* Secondary prevention after a non-haemorrhagic stroke or transient ischaemic attack: for at least 2 years after the stroke.

Usual dosage

* 200 mg (slow-release tablets) twice a day.

Side effects, contraindications, and precautions

The oral form is generally well tolerated, although some patients develop headaches and hot flushes.

Anticoagulants

Anticoagulants block specific blood proteins that are normally involved in the coagulation process. The effect on blood coagulation is stronger than that of antiplatelet agents and the risks of bleeding are higher. Therefore anticoagulants are reserved for conditions in which a strong inhibition of the clotting process is essential. Anticoagulants can be given by injection when a quick onset of action is needed or orally in chronic stable conditions. Their effect and use are monitored and checked using specific blood tests.

Injectable anticoagulants

These are almost always for hospital use and are only briefly discussed here as a reference.

Unfractionated heparin (generally known as heparin)

This is usually given by intravenous continuous infusion. The daily dose is weight-adjusted and the effect and safety are regularly checked by a specific blood test called APTT. As an inpatient, you may be given heparin in the following situations:

- pulmonary embolism
- deep vein thrombosis
- if you are bed-ridden or with limited mobility
- in the acute phase of a myocardial infarction
- selected cases of acute coronary syndromes.

Low-molecular-weight heparin (LMWH)

This is generally given subcutaneously once or twice a day. The daily dose is also weight-adjusted, but there is no need to check the effect. Since LMWH products (daltaparin, enoxiparin) are easier to administer, they are frequently and increasingly used instead of unfractionated heparin with similar effectiveness.

Oral anticoagulants

Initially used as rodenticides ('rat poison') in the 1940s, oral anticoagulants were introduced in clinical practice in the 1950s. The American President Dwight Eisenhower was one of the first and most famous cardiac patients to be treated with warfarin after a heart attack. Oral anticoagulants induce a sustained inhibition of blood coagulation by interfering with the metabolism of vitamin K (a normal component of diet, found mainly in green leafy vegetables). In contrast with the injectable agents discussed above, they are intended for long-term use in otherwise active individuals. The most widely used agent is warfarin.

Indications

- Patients with mechanical prosthetic cardiac valves: unlimited period.
- Selected cases of atrial fibrillation: as long as the problem is active.

109

- Patients with thrombi (clots) in the left ventricle, generally following a heart attack: for variable periods, possibly unlimited.
- Selected cases of severe cardiac failure: for variable periods, possibly unlimited.
- After pulmonary embolism or deep vein thrombosis: for variable periods, possibly unlimited.

Usual dosage

This is extremely variable and is guided by blood tests. The following numbers are for guidance only: 5–10 mg/day for a few days as loading, followed by 2.5–5 mg/day as maintenance.

Blood testing for warfarin treatment

A blood test called the international normalized ratio (INR) is used to ensure that the warfarin dosage provides the desired level of anticoagulation, without excessive risk of bleeding. The higher the INR, the stronger is the anticoagulant effect. At the beginning of the treatment, the INR has to be checked quite frequently, i.e. two or three times a week. As the INR stabilizes and the 'response pattern' of an individual patient becomes apparent, the frequency of INR checks may gradually be reduced to once a week and then once a month. The appropriate dose and frequency of INR checking may need to be reassessed whenever there is a change in your diet or concurrent medication or if you have an acute illness.

A healthy untreated individual with a balanced diet is expected to have a spontaneous INR of 0.8–1.2. The therapeutic range for most indications is 2–3, and the range for high-risk conditions and patients with a mechanical cardiac valve is 2.5–3.5. It should be noted that in real life some fluctuations out of the target range are unavoidable; however, unless they are persistent and excessive, they are generally of little clinical consequence.

Side effects, contraindications, and precautions

The main concern in patients taking warfarin is bleeding complications. However, this risk can be minimized if the following precautions are taken.

- Good INR monitoring routines exist (the risk of bleeding becomes significant at INR >4.5).
- Anticoagulants are not used or, if this is unavoidable, strict monitoring routines and precautions are in place with:
  - advanced age and general frailty
  - documented history of gastrointestinal bleeding/active disease
  - uncontrolled hypertension
  - recurrent falls
  - expected poor compliance with prescribed doses and INR monitoring
  - excess alcohol intake.

Other side effects, which occur rarely, are hair loss (reversible) and skin rash.

Warfarin is contraindicated in pregnancy since it can induce fetal malformations. Women taking warfarin who intend to become pregnant should consult their doctor. Breastfeeding is probably safe while taking warfarin, although medical advice should be sought.

Practical advice for patients taking warfarin

◆ Keep a record of your last INR values and doses taken (you may be provided with a notebook by your GP or anticoagulation monitoring clinic) and bring it with you whenever you are seen in a hospital or in your GP surgery.

◆ Consider having a medical bracelet or card indicating that you take warfarin. This can be extremely useful if you are involved in an accident or need urgent surgery.

◆ Avoid intense activities or sports that may result in injuries.

◆ Be careful to avoid even minor injuries.

◆ Contact your doctor if you develop new spontaneous bleeding, even minor, and consider 'skipping' a dose until you receive medical advice.

◆ Present to the nearest A&E department if you have more severe bleeding, such as vomiting blood, if you develop a severe headache, or if you are involved in an accident or a fall and hit your head, even if there is no evidence of bleeding.

◆ Be aware that drastic and prolonged diet changes can change your warfarin requirements. Green leafy vegetables, such as spinach, broccoli, lettuce, Brussels sprouts, cabbage, and cauliflower, are rich in vitamin K and may counteract the effects of warfarin, while carrots, potatoes, cucumbers, and eggplants (aubergines) have a low vitamin K content. Neither group should be avoided, but the vegetable content of your diet should be kept more or less constant. Vitamin and even herbal supplements can also interact with warfarin. Consult your doctor or pharmacist.

◆ Many prescription and over-the-counter drugs can interfere with warfarin, either increasing or decreasing its effect. Among frequently used drugs, painkillers, aspirin, antibiotics, and amiodarone can interfere with warfarin or potentiate its effects. In fact, the list of medications with possible interactions is so long that a rule of thumb is always to seek advice from your doctor or pharmacist before taking a new drug for a prolonged period. All that is needed in most cases is a period of more frequent monitoring of INR and dose adjustment.

Warfarin before planned surgery or dental work

Some procedures will require total cessation of warfarin and bringing the INR to 'physiological' levels, while others may be performed with a lower INR than is effective, although not necessarily in the normal range. The INR may require a few days to normalize after stopping warfarin. According to the indication for which you take warfarin, your doctor may decide to use heparin as a 'bridge' from the moment the INR has normalized until your surgery is performed, and then again when warfarin is restarted until the INR reaches again the target level. Good communication between your doctor and the doctor performing the procedure is essential.

Warfarin before emergency surgery

When unexpected surgery is needed or if bleeding occurs due to trauma, vitamin K and clotting factor transfusion are used for rapid reversal of the action of warfarin.

Nitrates

The use of nitroglycerin (glyceryl trinitrate (GTN)) in the relief of angina was pioneered in England in the nineteenth century and its ability to cause severe headache was noted at the same time. Today, nitroglycerine and isosorbide compounds are collectively known as nitrates and are used mainly in the symptomatic treatment of angina. They induce dilatation of coronary arteries, systemic arteries, and veins. They can be used either as short-acting agents to abort anginal attacks or as long-acting agents to prevent them. Nitrates may also be used in some cases of cardiac failure.

Indications

- To abort an anginal attack: short-acting agents, mainly GTN preparations
    - Tablets: for sublingual or buccal (placed between the lip and the gum) use
    - Sprays
- To prevent anginal attacks: long-acting agents
    - GTN preparations
        - Tablets
        - Transdermal patches
    - Isosorbide preparations

Nitrates are a symptomatic treatment and not a cure for angina. Therefore if your symptoms resolve after a revascularization procedure, a trial of stopping them can be made.

Usual dosage

- Short-acting agents
    - Sublingual tablets (0.3–0.6 mg) or sprays (0.4 mg per metered dose) are taken when symptoms begin and, owing to quick absorption, should

provide relief within a minute or so. A second dose may be taken after 5 minutes if needed.

◆ Long-acting agents

   ◆ The dose and the frequency depend on the specific preparation used. Tolerance can develop to repeated/prolonged effect, so a 'drug-free' interval (usually at night) is frequently advised when taking these agents.

Side effects, contraindications, and precautions

The most common side effect noted with nitrates is headache. This is severe enough to stop patients using the medication in only a minority of cases. Moreover, headache tends to diminish with continuous use. A more serious side effect is a sudden drop in blood pressure, resulting in dizziness or fainting. This is more likely to occur in the elderly, or with relative dehydration, although overall it is unpredictable. Using a small dose and, if possible, assuming a reclining position when the drug is taken for the first time is a good method of testing individual response.

There are some cardiac contraindications to the use of nitrates, such as severe aortic stenosis and hypertrophic cardiomyopathy. Short-acting preparations should be avoided with low blood pressure. The combination of nitrates with Viagra or similar products may induce dangerous drops in blood pressure. If you are taking nitrates and consider using Viagra, you should seek advice from your doctor. Nitrates are also contraindicated in closed-angle glaucoma; this is a less common variety of glaucoma and your ophthalmologist or GP should be able to advise you if necessary.

Practical advice for patients using nitrates

◆ Sublingual tablets have a short shelf-life after opening the bottle. Their efficacy may decrease so much that it is recommended that they are discarded after 8 weeks. If you are only an 'occasional' user, GTN spray may be a better alternative.

◆ Short-acting nitrates abort an angina attack but they do not, in any way, cure the disease. If you are intolerant of nitrates and your angina is clearly exercise related, just stopping your activity and waiting for the pain to subside may be acceptable for mild attacks.

◆ If the pain does not settle after two doses, it may be either non-anginal in nature (indigestion, muscular pain) or it may represent a more serious condition such as an impending heart attack, and you should consider seeking medical advice.

◆ Taking a sublingual tablet or spray just before engaging in a physical activity that you know will trigger your angina is a sensible way of preventing an anginal attack and allowing you to continue with your activities.

Other anti-anginal agents

Nicorandil

Nicorandil resembles nitrates in inducing coronary and systemic vasodilatation although its mechanism of action is more complex. Nicorandil is used mainly for the symptomatic treatment of angina, either in addition to nitrates or as an alternative when nitrates are not tolerated. It shares with the nitrates some possible side effects such as headache and flushing. A more specific, although rare, side effect is oral ulcerations. Usual doses are 10–20 mg twice a day.

Ivabradine

Ivabradine is a representative of a new class of drugs that act by specifically inhibiting the sinus node function and inducing bradycardia. This is beneficial in patients with exercise-induced angina; ivabradine resembles beta-blockers in this respect, but without the wider cardioprotective effects of the latter. At the present time, ivabradine has a quite narrow indication in patients with exercise-induced angina who cannot receive beta-blockers. The same precautions as for beta-blockers apply regarding possible excessive heart rate reduction. A more specific, although rare, side effect is visual disturbances, mainly luminous phenomena. As with some other drugs, consumption of grapefruit juice should be avoided as it may interfere with ivabradine metabolism and potentiate its actions. Usual doses are 2.5–7.5 mg twice a day.

Beta-blockers

In 1948, an American scientist, Raymond Ahlquist, introduced the concept of alpha- and beta-receptors to explain why the same catecholamines (substances present in blood and nerve endings) have either stimulating or inhibitory effects, depending on the target tissue or organ. Stimulation of beta-receptors can induce a wide array of responses such as increased heart rate and contractility (beta-1 effects), and vascular and bronchial relaxation (beta-2 effects). Following more than 10 years of research, the first beta-blocker for clinical use, propranolol, was invented by the Scottish scientist Sir James Black in 1964, opening a new era in the treatment of heart diseases. For this and other contributions to clinical pharmacology he was awarded the Nobel Prize for medicine in 1988. Today, beta-blockers comprise about 15 compounds that are central to the treatment of a variety of cardiovascular and some non-cardiac conditions. All beta-blockers share the main effects of what is known as beta-blockade:

- heart rate slowing
- blood pressure lowering
- myocardial contractile depression (not usually of clinical consequence)
- possible bronchoconstriction (of concern only in patients with asthma or bronchitis)
- peripheral vessel constriction (of concern only in patients with peripheral vascular disease or vasospastic conditions).

Indications

Beta-blockers are widely used in the treatment of various cardiovascular conditions, such as angina, hypertension, arrhythmias, and cardiac failure, or after a heart attack. In addition to the symptomatic benefits in angina, some arrhythmias, and heart failure, they lower mortality and the risk of further cardiac events in patients with decreased left ventricular function or after a heart attack. As a general rule, beta-blockers are given for long and possibly unlimited periods of time.

Beta-blockers are also occasionally used in some non-cardiac conditions: migraine, tremor hyperthyroidism, and glaucoma (local use).

Usual dosage

The available beta-blockers differ mainly in terms of duration of action and potency of non-cardiac effects, although the latter difference is less important at high doses. Your doctor will decide which beta-blocker is the most suitable for you. The most widely used beta-blockers and their usual dosage range are listed in Table 14.2. Individual response varies considerably, and the decrease in heart rate can be used to gauge whether the desired effect has been achieved. A resting heart rate of 50–55 beats/minute indicates good beta-blockade.

Side effects, contraindications, and precautions

Beta-blockers are generally well tolerated. Most side effects are direct consequences of their pharmacological actions and should be prevented by good patient selection and dose titration.

Slow heart rate

A certain degree of slowing of the heart rate is normal and in fact expected in patients taking beta-blockers. If well tolerated and not excessive, it should not be seen as a side effect. Precaution or total avoidance are recommended in patients with a spontaneous low heart rate, ECG evidence of being at risk of slow heart rate, or when other drugs with the potential of lowering the heart rate are taken.

Table 14.2 The most widely used beta-blockers

Propranolol	40–240 mg/day
Atenolol*†	25–100 mg/day
Bisoprolol*†	2.5–10 mg/day
Metoprolol†	100–200 mg/day
Carvedilol*	6.25–50 mg/day
Sotalol	80–320 mg/day

*Long-acting agents.
†Cardio-selective (fewer non-cardiac effects).

Hypotension

Beta-blockers can occasionally induce hypotension.

Bronchospasm

Beta-blockers are generally contraindicated in known asthmatic patients. Selective beta-blockers (see Table 14.2) can be tried, although their 'asthma-friendly' qualities are probably lost at high doses. Beta-blockers are not generally contraindicated in all lung conditions, but only in those with a clear bronchospastic component.

Peripheral vasoconstriction

Some patients will complain of 'cold extremities' while taking beta-blockers. They should be used with caution or avoided in patients with known vasospastic conditions or peripheral vascular disease.

Various non-cardiovascular effects

General fatigue, nightmares, sexual dysfunction, exacerbation of psoriasis, and dry eyes.

General precaution

Abrupt and persistent cessation of beta-blockers, especially if used at high dose and for a long time, can result in a sudden increase in heart rate and blood pressure (rebound phenomenon), accompanied by anxiety and possible worsening of cardiac symptoms. Any cessation of beta-blocker treatment has to be done gradually and while consulting with your doctor.

Calcium-channel blockers

Free motion of calcium ions through cell membranes is essential for muscle cell activation. Calcium-channel blockers are a group of agents that induce vasodilatation, decrease heart rate, and may depress cardiac contractility. Calcium-channel blockers can be subdivided into two groups according to their main effects:

- mainly vasodilators: nifedipine, amlodipine, felodipine
- able to slow the heart rate as well: verapamil, diltiazem.

Indications

The nifedipine–amlodipine–felodipine group is used when the main desired effect is vasodilatation. These drugs can be used in angina and are valuable anti-hypertensive agents.

The verapamil–diltiazem group is used when the main desired effect is slowing the heart rate. They are useful in the treatment and prophylaxis of some cardiac arrhythmias (atrial fibrillation, supraventricular tachycardia) and are a reasonable alternative to beta-blockers in selected patients with angina who will not tolerate the latter.

Usual dosage

◆ Nifedipine (long-acting compounds are preferred): 20–60 mg once daily

◆ Amlodipine: 5–10 mg once daily

◆ Felodipine: 2.5–10 mg once daily

◆ Verapamil: 40–120 mg three times a day (long-acting compounds are available)

◆ Diltiazem: 30–60 mg three times a day (long-acting compounds are available).

Side effects, contraindications, and precautions

As expected, the vasodilator group can induce headache and flushing. More specific to this group is the possible occurrence of leg oedema. Awareness of this side effect is important so that it will not be considered a sign of heart failure. Like other vasodilators, these calcium-channel blockers should be used cautiously or avoided in the presence of severe aortic stenosis.

Verapamil and diltiazem may cause bradycardia and, as for beta-blockers, they should be used cautiously or avoided in patients with a spontaneously slow heart rate or at risk of developing excessive bradycardia. Unlike beta-blockers, they are contraindicated in patients with decreased left ventricular contractility. More specifically, verapamil may induce constipation. Leg oedema is less likely, but is still possible with these products.

Digoxin

Digoxin (a compound extracted from the foxglove) has been almost synonymous with standard treatment of heart failure since the Scottish physician William Withering advocated its use in 1776. Digoxin has a proven effect of strengthening heart contractility and, in certain conditions, slowing the heart rate. However, despite its historical credentials, the exact place of digoxin in the management of heart failure is still under discussion. Unlike beta-blockers and ACE inhibitors that are used in the treatment of heart failure for both symptomatic relief and to improve long-term outcome, digoxin provides symptomatic relief only.

Indications

Generally agreed possible indications for digoxin are congestive heart failure with atrial fibrillation and congestive heart failure that is still symptomatic despite use of other treatments. Digoxin is also used to control the heart rate in atrial fibrillation.

Usual dosage

Frequently, digoxin is started with a loading dose which is continued with a maintenance dosage of 62.5–250 mcg/day, depending on age, renal function, and heart rate response.

Side effects, contraindications, and precautions

Because of its potential to lower the heart rate, digoxin is subject to same precautions and contraindications as for beta-blockers and calcium-channel blockers. Severe bradycardia, rhythm disturbances, and non-cardiac phenomena such as vomiting and, rarely, coloured vision are all possible side effects and can happen alone or in combination. These complications, occasionally described as 'digoxin toxicity', may be secondary to documented overdosage but may also occur with usual dosage in patients who have been taking digoxin for a long time. Elderly patients and those with impaired renal function are more at risk of developing digoxin side effects. The following factors can trigger or worsen digoxin toxicity:

- dehydration
- worsening of renal function
- low blood potassium levels (possibly secondary to use of diuretics)
- concomitant intake of other medications that potentiate digoxin effects or raise its blood levels.

General precautions and advice for patients taking digoxin

- Digoxin blood level monitoring
  - Blood level monitoring is not routinely used but can occasionally be requested by your doctor to guide digoxin dosage. However, digoxin toxicity is also possible at 'normal' levels.
- Interaction with other drugs
  - Some medications (verapamil, amiodarone) may potentiate digoxin effects or can increase its blood levels. Consult with your doctor before starting a new cardiovascular drug.

Diuretics

Diuretics promote excretion of water and sodium through the kidneys (diuresis), increasing the volume of urine. They are frequently used to treat hypertension and are crucial in the management of symptomatic heart failure. From a patient's perspective, there are three main groups of diuretics.

Diuretics with moderate effect and long-term action (thiazide diuretics)

These diuretics are used in mild hypertension, especially in the elderly, in patients of African descent, and in mild cases of heart failure. For these indications, higher doses are generally not more effective and their use is fraught with an increased incidence of side effects. They are not effective in the presence of renal failure.

- Usual dosage:
  - Bendroflumetazide: 2.5 mg once a day

- Side effects, contraindications, and precautions
  - Thiazide diuretics are generally well tolerated at low doses. With increased doses there is a risk of low potassium levels and an increase in glucose and lipid levels. Even with low doses, occasional blood checks are useful with long-term treatment.

Diuretics with a powerful effect and short-term action (loop diuretics)

These diuretics are used with more severe cases of heart failure. They are also efficient in the presence of renal failure (at higher doses), have a short time of onset and of activity, and therefore can be repeated if necessary. For increased effect, they can be combined with thiazides, and in severe cases can also be given intravenously.

- Usual dosage (long-term, oral treatment)
  - Furosemide: 40–80 mg daily or more
  - Bumetanide: 1–3 mg daily or more
- Side effects, contraindications, and precautions
  - The risks of electrolyte disturbances (low sodium, potassium, and magnesium levels) are higher than with thiazides because of the more intense effect and the higher doses used. Prolonged use of high doses may worsen renal failure. Deafness and vertigo can occur after prolonged use of large intravenous doses.

Potassium-sparing diuretics

Chronic depletion of the body potassium stores is a concern with prolonged use of both thiazide and loop diuretics. Low potassium levels are associated with an increased risk of cardiac arrhythmias. Further potassium loss is promoted by aldosterone, a naturally occurring hormone that is excessively released in patients with severe oedema and acts at renal level to retain water and sodium at the expense of potassium. Anti-aldosterone compounds are used to counteract this effect and thus to preserve potassium stores. On their own, the potassium-sparing agents are weak diuretics, but when combined with either thiazides or loop diuretics they can potentiate their action and preserve potassium levels. A few compounds, with slightly different mechanisms of action, are available. The most widely used is spironolactone, which acts by directly opposing the action of aldosterone.

- Spironolactone indications and usual dosage
  - For potassium-sparing effect in association with other diuretics: 25–50 mg/day
  - For diuresis potentiation in patients with severe oedema due to cardiac failure or cirrhosis: 100–200 mg/day
  - In selected patients with decreased ventricular contractility after a heart attack: 25 mg/day

♦ Side effects, contraindications, and precautions

  ♦ Potassium-sparing diuretics should not be given together with potassium supplements, and caution is recommended when they are associated with other drugs that can raise potassium levels. Pre-existing renal failure and baseline elevated potassium levels are a relative contraindication, and caution or total avoidance are recommended in these patients. Spironolactone has some specific side effects such as gynaecomastia (growth in breast size in male patients).

Angiotensin-converting enzyme (ACE) inhibitors

Angiotensin II is a strong vasoconstrictor which is produced by the activation (by a converting enzyme) of its precursor angiotensin I, a compound resulting from the interaction of renin (produced by the kidney) with angiotensinogen (produced by the liver). Inhibition of the converting enzyme by ACE inhibitors results in lowering of the blood pressure. However, it was quickly found that, since angiotensin II has numerous biological effects beyond vasoconstriction, ACE inhibitors have more complex and beneficial actions than just hypertension control. Indeed, they are credited with protective effects on patients with diabetes, after a heart attack, or with decreased ventricular contractility, and, like beta-blockers, they have had a major impact on the modern management of many cardiovascular conditions. The association of hypertension with diabetes or heart failure or a previous myocardial infarction is a strong argument for the use of ACE inhibitors.

Indications

ACE inhibitors are widely used in patients

♦ with arterial hypertension
♦ with heart failure
♦ after a heart attack
♦ with renal complications of diabetes.

Usual dosage

Following the first available ACE inhibitors, captopril and enalapril, numerous other products have been developed. They all share the same class effects and differ mainly in dosage and tolerability, although the differences tend to be minimal between compounds developed after captopril. Also, more data are available for some ACE inhibitors regarding cardiovascular protective effects and this may influence prescription practice.

♦ Captopril: 25–50 mg twice a day
♦ Enalapril: 10–20 mg once a day
♦ Ramipril: 2.5–10 mg once a day
♦ Perindopril: 2–8 mg once a day
♦ Lisinopril: 10–20 mg once a day

Side effects, contraindications, and precautions

ACE inhibitors are generally very well tolerated. About 10% of patients (more frequently women) will develop a dry cough that may be irritating enough to warrant cessation of treatment and use of an alternative drug (see below). A rare side effect is an allergic reaction with oedema of the face, lips, and tongue. ACE inhibitors occasionally cause deterioration of renal function; this happens mainly in patients with severe narrowing of the renal arteries, but caution should be exerted in the elderly, patients with pre-existing renal failure, and those concomitantly treated with a high dose of diuretics or anti-inflammatory drugs. Renal function and electrolyte levels should be checked at baseline and after starting the treatment. Severe hypotension is rare with ACE inhibitors but can occur with concomitant dehydration or intense use of diuretics.

Angiotensin receptor blockers (ARBs)

ARBs are very similar to ACE inhibitors and they have practically the same indications, although licenses may differ for individual agents. They have a slightly different mechanism of action (by blocking angiotensin II receptors) and as result are much less likely to induce cough or allergic reactions. Although they are probably as effective as ACE inhibitors and can be chosen as first-line treatment for the same indications, in practice they are frequently reserved for those patients who develop cough while taking ACE inhibitors. Except for cough, the spectrum of side effects and necessary precautions is similar to that of ACE inhibitors. As for ACE inhibitors, several compounds are available.

Usual dosage

- Losartan: 25–50 mg once daily
- Candesartan: 4–8 mg once daily
- Irbesartan: 75–300 mg once daily
- Valsartan: 40–160 mg once daily
- Telmisartan: 40–80 mg once daily.

Alpha-blockers

These drugs are effective anti-hypertensives, inducing vasodilatation by blocking the peripheral alpha-receptors. They are useful adjuvants when first- and second-line anti-hypertensive are not enough to achieve good control. They may be a good option in elderly males with prostatism since they relax the bladder neck and facilitate micturition. The main concern with these agents is postural hypotension. Elderly patients should be instructed to avoid dehydration and sudden standing. Also, treatment should be initiated with small doses to test individual response.

Usual dosage

- Doxazosin: 1–8 mg daily
- Prazosin: 0.5–1mg three times a day.

Centrally acting anti-hypertensives

Once the mainstay of anti-hypertensive treatment, these agents (clonidine, methyldopa, monoxidine) are rarely used today because of the availability of newer agents with fewer side effects. They act by inhibiting the central nervous system activity responsible for vascular tone and blood pressure. They may be used in cases of hypertension that is resistant to the usual drugs. Because of its safety record methyldopa is used for hypertension in pregnancy.

Anti-arrhythmics

Various agents are available for the treatment of rhythm disturbances, some of which are for restricted specialist use. The general 'philosophy' of using anti-arrhythmic drugs has changed over the last 20 years (see Chapter 7). Some arrhythmias have been found to be less dangerous than the potential side effects of some anti-arrhythmic drugs, and strategies have been developed to identify high-risk patients and use procedures or devices to prevent arrhythmia recurrence or major arrhythmic complications, rather than prescribing anti-arrhythmic medication. Paradoxically, in some categories of patients, anti-arrhythmics can increase the risk of arrhythmia. The decision to use an anti-arrhythmic agent is a highly individualized one which takes into account the benefits of suppressing the arrhythmia, the expected side effects, and the overall 'risk profile' of a given patient. It is beyond the scope of this book to detail the characteristics of all available anti-arrhythmics; instead, short summaries of the anti-arrhythmic agents that the average cardiac patient is likely to be prescribed are presented.

Beta-blockers (see pp. 114–116)

Beta-blockers are relatively weak anti-arrhythmics. They can be used for mild cases of ventricular and supraventricular arrhythmia. Alternatively, they are used to slow the heart rate of patients with atrial fibrillation.

Calcium-channel blockers (see pp. 116–117)

Verapamil and diltiazem are also relatively weak anti-arrhythmics, although they can be useful in supraventricular arrhythmias. Unlike beta-blockers, they are contraindicated in the presence of reduced ventricular contractility and have almost no place in the treatment of ventricular arrhythmia.

Flecainide and propafenone

Flecainide (usual dose: 100–400 mg/day) and propafenone (usual dose: 450–900 mg/day) are effective anti-arrhythmics used in the treatment of supraventricular and selected ventricular arrhythmia. They are formally contraindicated in patients with left ventricular dysfunction; propafenone is also relatively contraindicated in patients with chronic obstructive lung disease. Both can worsen pre-existing heart failure, bradycardia, or arrhythmias in susceptible patients. As a rule they should be initiated by a specialist cardiologist.

Amiodarone

Amiodarone is probably the most effective anti-arrhythmic agent available, with a spectrum of action covering both supraventricular and ventricular arrhythmias. Unlike other anti-arrhythmics, it is very rarely associated with significant cardiac side effects and can even be given to patients with advanced heart failure. The limiting factor in the use of amiodarone is an array of possible non-cardiac side effects and complications: hypo- or hyperthyroidism, gastric intolerance, visual disturbances, skin discolouration, hepatic toxicity, and lung toxicity (potentially severe). Most of these complications are reversible. However, the overall tolerance of amiodarone is good, although the benefit–risk ratio should be carefully assessed in all patients, especially when long-term treatment is contemplated. Baseline thyroid, liver, and lung assessments are recommended before initiation of therapy, followed by periodic (once or twice a year) liver and thyroid function tests. Amiodarone is generally started with a loading regimen, followed by a maintenance dose of 200 mg/day.

Sotalol

Sotalol is a special beta-blocker with distinct anti-arrhythmic properties. It can be used for both ventricular and supraventricular arrhythmias, with an efficacy close to that of amiodarone, and it is a reasonable choice in patients with normal hearts who also have angina. However, unlike amiodarone, sotalol is not suitable for patients with heart failure and may worsen or induce ventricular arrhythmias. Patients with renal failure or with a tendency to hypokalaemia may be particularly at risk. Usual doses are 80–320 mg/day.

 Frequently Asked Questions

Grapefruit and medications

Q: I always thought of grapefruit juice as of one of the healthiest natural juices. But now a friend told me that she read in a newspaper that grapefruit juice can dangerously interact with some drugs. I have just started taking a new high blood pressure tablet. Should I avoid grapefruit juice now?

A: Grapefruit is indeed considered a very healthy natural product because of its low calorie and high vitamin C and antioxidant content. In the 1980s, grapefruit juice was incidentally found to raise the circulating levels of some drugs by blocking an enzyme found in the liver and intestine. Of interest for cardiac patients, such interactions have been described for statins, some calcium-channel blockers, and amiodarone. The effects of grapefruit juice on the metabolism of affected drugs can last for up to 72 hours.

Of note, these are mainly experimental data and the real clinical impact and risk are still unclear. As things stand now, patients taking drugs known to be affected by grapefruit should refrain from its consumption, and if in doubt consult with their doctor or pharmacist.

Painkillers and heart disease

Q: I have diabetes and hypertension and had bypass surgery a few years ago. I do have some bad pains in my knees and have been diagnosed with osteoarthritis. I really need some painkillers, otherwise I am barely able to walk on some days. I have heard a few 'horror stories' about getting a stomach ulcer or even being at a risk of a heart attack from using painkillers, so I really don't know what to do now.

A: Occasional use of painkillers (analgesics) is generally of no concern, but their long-term use does raise some issues. Most painkillers also have an anti-inflammatory action, and act by inhibiting two enzymes (COX-1 and COX-2) involved in the inflammatory response, and they are collectively known as non-steroidal anti-inflammatory drugs (NSAIDs). The most widely used agents, such as diclofenac, ibuprofen naproxen, and indomethacin, may induce gastric irritation. The risk increases with advanced age, long period of use, and high doses, and it is of particular concern in cardiac patients who are already taking aspirin. NSAIDs can also worsen renal function in patients at risk (diabetics, hypertensives, or those with pre-existing renal disease). A particular concern exists about a more recent class of NSAIDs, the coxibs (celecoxib, etoricoxib), which have been specifically developed to minimize the risk of gastric ulceration by selectively inhibiting the COX-2 enzyme only. However, it has been found that their use is associated with an increased risk of cardiovascular events, possibly related to their lack of inhibition of blood platelets, which are inhibited to a certain extent by non-selective NSAIDs. Therefore if you are a cardiac patient or have risk factors for cardiovascular disease or pre-existing renal disease or a history of ulcer, you may consider the following.

⧫ Consider using paracetamol as a painkiller. Alone or combined with codeine in various over-the-counter preparations, paracetamol is a well-tolerated and effective analgesic that may allow you either to avoid a standard NSAID or to reduce its frequency or dosage.

⧫ If you have to use NSAIDS:

  ⧫ Use the minimum effective dose and the shortest possible course. Take 'breaks' if possible (paracetamol can help).

  ⧫ Consider some gastric protection drugs if you use aspirin as well (seek advice from your doctor).

◆ As a rule, do not use coxibs unless the indication is clear and you do not have coronary disease or its risk factors.

When should I take my tablets?

Q: Since I had my heart attack, I take quite a lot of medications. Should I take them together or at different times?

A: Most cardiac medications are taken once daily and their timing is quite flexible. Very few have specific timing indications, such as statins which should be taken in the evening. Others, such as beta-blockers and nitrates, are better taken in the morning to give maximum anti-anginal protection during daily activities. Some patients find that taking aspirin after the main meal is better tolerated. Patients taking diuretics may decide to avoid an evening schedule, so that they will not have to wake up at night to pass urine. If multiple anti-hypertensive medications are taken, spacing them out is a good idea to avoid sudden blood pressure drops and ensure a uniform blood pressure control. Finally, some patients may decide that an 'all of them together' approach is more convenient, while others may go for a 'morning–evening' schedule. The scenarios described above should help you to decide which medication schedule is most suitable to your particular needs.

Q: Sometimes I am in a rush, and I only have time for a cup of coffee. Does it make any difference if I take my tablets on an empty stomach or after a meal?

A: In most cases it does not make much difference, but some medications may have different absorption or may be less tolerated depending on whether they are taken on an empty stomach or with food. The best routine is to follow the instructions on each medication leaflet. If in doubt, consult your pharmacist.

Q: What if I forget to take a dose?

A: Most cardiac drugs have a prolonged action time and forgetting a dose is unlikely to be significant. The general principle is to continue as scheduled, although for some medications you may want to bring the next dose earlier. In no case should you 'make it up' and double the next dose.

Q: I take so many tablets for my heart condition, my diabetes, and my bronchitis. How do I know that there are no unwanted interactions between all these medications?

A: The odds for significant interactions are low and, generally speaking, it is the responsibility of your doctor and your pharmacist to ensure that this does not happen. When you are prescribed a new medication by someone who is not your regular doctor, it is a good idea to make sure that he/she is aware of your present medications. Also, you should consult with the pharmacist whenever you take an over-the-counter drug.

Various brands

Q: I have been taking cholesterol and blood pressure tablets for many years, but of late I have noticed different names on some tablet boxes. Some of my friends have noticed the same change. I have questioned my pharmacist and he reassured me that these are different brands of the same product and that I have no reason to worry. Nevertheless I am concerned as I have always been told how important it was to follow my prescription strictly.

A: Each new drug is initially manufactured and distributed under a registered name by the pharmacological company that developed it. Once their exclusive patent expires, other manufacturers may produce the same drug and market it under different names, and your medical organization may decide to use any of them, based on price and reliability of supply considerations. The fact that their products are now on the market means that they have satisfied all the strict requirements of the regulatory bodies regarding quality and equivalence with the original product, so your pharmacist was right and you should not be concerned. A different issue may arise if you are switched to an equivalent but not identical drug, such as a different beta-blocker or ACE inhibitor. Usually there is a good clinical reason for your doctor to do this, but you can ask him/her for clarification if you are concerned.

15

Pacemakers and related devices

> **→ Key Points**
>
> ◆ Low heart rate (bradycardia) may result in dizziness or even loss of consciousness.
>
> ◆ There is no effective medical treatment for symptomatic bradycardia.
>
> ◆ Pacemakers are electronic devices that stimulate the heart to avoid drops in heart rate.
>
> ◆ Special pacemakers and related devices are used to control arrhythmias and improve symptoms in patients with heart failure.

Pacemakers

Bradyarrhythmias have been discussed in Chapter 7. A heart rate slower than 60 beats/minute is formally defined as bradycardia, but the point at which an individual becomes symptomatic varies very much: some patients may experience symptoms at heart rates of 40–50 beats/minute, while others may tolerate heart rates in the range 30–40 beats/minute surprisingly well.

In addition, young athletes tend to have well-tolerated low heart rates in the range that would probably be symptomatic in most individuals. In affected individuals, bradycardia or bradyarrhythmias can occur intermittently only, making the diagnosis difficult, since between episodes the patient is asymptomatic and has a normal heart rate. Typical symptoms possibly associated with slow heart rate are:

◆ dizziness

◆ syncope and presyncope.

Other possible symptoms associated with bradycardia are:

◆ fatigue (occasionally exertional, since there is no appropriate heart rate rise with exercise)

◆ progressive cardiac failure.

Although slow heart rates have to be documented for a formal diagnosis, their occurrence may be suspected from the clinical presentation and tests such as ECG tape recording may further clarify the diagnosis. Alternatively, suggestive symptoms and some specific ECG changes may be enough to decide that this is the problem even if the actual bradycardia is not documented. The only practical answer for patients with persistent or recurrent symptomatic bradycardia or whose ECG shows risk features is implantation of a permanent pacemaker. Pacemakers are devices consisting of a self-contained non-rechargeable battery and electronic circuitry which generates electric impulses that are delivered to the heart through electrodes that are generally placed in the right heart cavities. Pacemakers brought a major revolution in the outcome and treatment of otherwise untreatable conditions and returned scores of patients to a normal life. After a few trials with bulky external devices, the first implantable pacemakers were inserted in the late 1950s. Their design and miniaturization improved constantly and modern pacemakers are small unobtrusive devices (Figure 15.1) with highly sophisticated detection and response capabilities to cover various bradyarrhythmias.

How are pacemakers implanted?

Under local anaesthesia and using a small incision, a 'pocket' is made under the skin, generally below the left clavicle. The pacemaker box is placed within

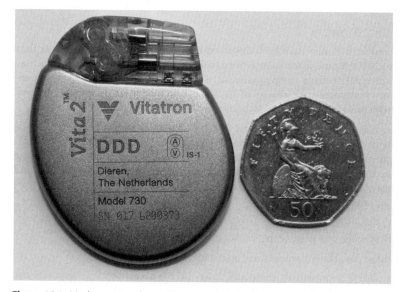

Figure 15.1 Modern pacemaker. A 50 pence coin is displayed as well for size comparison.

the subcutaneous fat tissue pocket and electrodes are advanced, using X-ray guidance, through the subclavian and the superior vena cava veins to the right atrium and the right ventricle (Figure 15.2). The whole procedure should not take more than an hour for standard pacemakers, although occasionally it may take longer. In uncomplicated cases, you should expect to go home the next day after a few checks of the device. Most hospitals will provide you with a leaflet explaining all that you should know about the procedure.

Risks and complications of the procedure

Pacemaker implantation is a small low-risk surgical procedure involving vascular access, but, as for any intervention, some complications can occur

- puncture of the lung and leaking of air around it (pneumothorax)
- infection
- local bleeding.

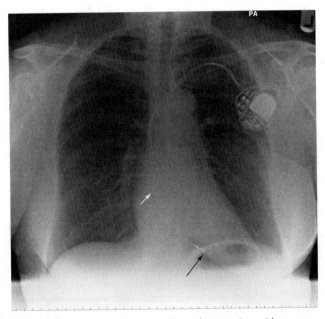

Figure 15.2 Typical appearance of a chest radiograph in a patient with a permanent pacemaker. The tip of one electrode is located in the right ventricle (black arrow) and the tip of the second electrode is located in the right atrium (white arrow). Both electrodes originate from the pacemaker box and follow the left subclavian vein and the superior vena cava to reach the heart.

However, the odds for any of these complications are very low, and in the unlikely event that they do occur, they are immediately recognized and appropriately treated.

How do pacemakers work?

The pacemaker senses any drop in heart rate below a pre-defined value, and when this happens it starts stimulating the heart. The first-generation pacemakers sensed and paced the right ventricle only ('single-chamber pacemakers') and had a rather crude 'all or nothing' response, whereby they always responded with a fixed rate without taking into account what the optimal heart rate would be or the cause of the pulse drop. Improved models (also known as VVI pacemakers) are still occasionally used with limited indications in patients with low levels of activity or persistent atrial arrhythmias. Most pacemakers in current use (known as dual-chamber or DDD pacemakers) have two electrodes to monitor and pace both the right atrium and the right ventricle as needed. They have sophisticated sensing and pacing algorithms allowing them to pace either the atrium or the ventricle, depending on the mechanism of the bradycardia, and ensuring that a physiological delay is maintained between the atrial and ventricular contraction. Modern pacemakers have motion-sensing capabilities and are able to vary the pacing rate according to the patient's level of activity. They can also be programmed to deliver a lower heart rate at night.

What happens after the pacemaker implantation?

After a very short recovery period (few days), you can expect to return to your normal activities. You should be given a 'pacemaker identity card' detailing the type of the pacemaker, the implantation date, and its basic settings. You will enter a pacemaker follow-up programme to cover the unlikely occurrence of pacemaker malfunction and in order to detect the need for battery replacement in good time. Occasionally, some of the parameters have to be reprogrammed to reflect possible changes in your clinical condition. If the symptoms for which you underwent pacemaker implantation, such as dizziness or fainting, recur, you should alert your doctor so that the pacemaker can be checked. Many pacemakers have a 'memory' function, so that if you have significant arrhythmias or bradycardias and the pacemaker does not respond appropriately, this can be documented. Overall, however, pacemakers are very reliable devices with many built-in safety features, and the odds of technical failure are very low. The usual battery life is 8–10 years, and when it reaches its end 'warning signs' will be picked up at your routine follow-up pacemaker check. There is no way in which a pacemaker will suddenly stop working because of an empty battery so, as long as you regularly attend your clinic appointments, you should not be concerned about this. In order to ensure maximum fluid tightness, the pacemaker is constructed as a single sealed block, so that the battery cannot be removed. When it approaches the end of its lifetime, the whole device has to be removed and replaced with a new one. As the electrodes remain in place, this is a very low-risk and straightforward small surgical procedure.

Possible long-term complications

Generally, there are very few long-term complications in patients with permanent pacemakers. However, the following are of possible concern.

- Partial electrode fracture: electrode mechanical failures are extremely rare these days and are usually picked up at pacemaker check-up visits.

- Electrode displacement: there is a small risk of electrode displacement during the first 4–6 weeks after the procedure which may be related to not avoiding vigorous arm motion during this period.

- Skin erosion: this is less of a concern with modern small low-profile devices, but it can happen in very 'skinny' individuals with very little subcutaneous tissue.

- Infection: there is a small risk of infection either after the implantation or, occasionally, much later. Warning signs are local signs of infection at the site of the pocket or otherwise unexplained prolonged or recurrent fever. If this the case, you should contact your GP or your pacemaker clinic as soon as possible.

Special pacemakers and similar devices

For many years, the only indication for pacemakers was to treat bradyarrhythmias. However, technological and developmental advances have expanded the use of pacemaker-based devices to the treatment of selected cases of arrhythmias and heart failure.

Defibrillators

Patients who survive major heart attacks or with some genetically determined conditions may be at risk of life-threatening arrhythmias. No drug regimen, including specific anti-arrhythmic medication, has been found which significantly diminishes this risk. The life-saving effect of external cardioversion in patients with ventricular tachycardia or fibrillation has been known since the 1960s. However, early defibrillators were bulky devices, and the idea of a small implantable defibrillator was initially dismissed as impractical. It took the perseverance of Dr Michael Mirowski, an Israeli cardiologist working in the USA, to promote this concept, and as a result the first internal defibrillator was surgically implanted at Johns Hopkins Hospital, Baltimore, in 1980, ushering in an era of hope for patients at risk of sudden death. Current implantable cardioverter–defibrillators (ICDs) are sophisticated devices, which are slightly larger than regular pacemakers but inserted in the same way. As well as having all the functions of a pacemaker, ICDs detect threatening arrhythmias and deliver an internal shock which results in resumption of a normal rhythm. Their life-saving abilities have been proven beyond any doubt by many studies, and today defibrillators are routinely implanted in patients at risk.

Accepted indications for defibrillators

Indications for ICD implantation may vary slightly, with guidelines being more flexible or stricter in different countries, but the following represent the generally accepted straightforward indications.

◆ Survivors of large myocardial infarctions with either syncopal episodes or documented life-threatening arrhythmias, or other high-risk features.

◆ Successfully resuscitated sudden death due to documented arrhythmia when no immediate treatable cause was confirmed, irrespective of the baseline heart disease.

◆ Patients with various cardiomyopathies or genetic electrical abnormalities, such as long-QT syndrome, who satisfy high-risk criteria.

Biventricular pacemakers

Patients with severe heart failure frequently have an abnormal propagation of the electrical impulses within the myocardium that further worsens the strength of the ventricular contraction. It has been shown that this abnormal electrical activation can be corrected by electrical stimulation of both the left and right ventricles, and not just the right ventricle as for standard pacing. As a result, the left ventricle contractility improves. Therefore these pacemakers are called biventricular, although technically the electrode for the left ventricle is placed not within the ventricle but in a coronary vein that courses along the ventricular wall. Overall, the implantation procedure is more demanding and takes a longer time than for a standard pacemaker. Biventricular pacemakers are a valuable tool for improving the symptoms and survival of selected patients with severe heart failure. Devices with both biventricular pacing and defibrillation capabilities are also available.

 Frequently Asked Questions

Q: A few months ago I started to complain of dizzy spells. My doctor found that I had a low pulse and I had a pacemaker implanted. Apparently nothing else was wrong with my heart and since then I am perfectly well and fit. Are there any limitations that, nevertheless, I should be aware of? Can I move my arm freely and lift heavy weights?

A: You are expected to have a completely normal life with no limitations, although you will be advised to avoid strenuous activities, especially involving the upper part of the body, and avoid lifting the arm on the side of the pacemaker above shoulder level for about 6 weeks, until the electrodes are well stabilized.

Q: How do I know that my pacemaker is working properly? Am I supposed to feel anything?

A: If you had frequent symptoms before pacemaker implantation, their disappearance is a good indication that the pacemaker is working properly. Depending on how the pacemaker is programmed and the reason for which it has been implanted, some patients may occasionally detect its activity. As a rule, however, the pacemaker works silently in the background and you are not expected to feel anything. An obvious exception is when a shock is delivered by an ICD system, since this is always unmistakably perceived by the patient. For objective testing, pacemakers are routinely checked at least once a year in pacemaker clinics.

Q: Is there any problem with home appliances, electronic devices, or security checks at airports?

A: Pacemakers can be influenced by electromagnetic interference. However, the safety features of modern pacemakers and the manufacturing standards with which all modern equipment has to comply mean that pacemakers are safe in most home and working environments, and there is no concern in using most common appliances including computers, TV sets, remote control units, microwave ovens, electric razors and toothbrushes, and similar devices. Mobile phones are safe, although the manufacturers recommend that they should be kept no closer than 6 inches from the pacemaker and that you should use the ear on the opposite part of the body to the device. Larger but still perfectly convenient 'safety' distances (12–24 inches) are recommended for devices or tools generating high-intensity electromagnetic fields, such as power tools, and lawn mowers. Going through security archways is safe, although you should inform the security personnel (have your pacemaker card with you). The use of security wands should be limited or avoided altogether in the proximity of the pacemaker, and a hand search is preferable.

Q: I had my pacemaker implanted a year ago and now I need to have surgery for my gallbladder. Is this going to be a problem? What about the various tests that I may need prior to the operation?

A: If you have a pacemaker and need to undergo surgery, you have to inform the surgeon because some precautions are necessary to allow the use of techniques to stop bleeding, such as electrocautery and diathermy. Ultrasound scans, X-ray examinations, and CT scans are perfectly safe but, as a rule, MR scans are contraindicated al though this may change in the future.

If you need more detailed information about your pacemaker, you can ask your cardiologist or the pacemaker clinic or you can use the website of the manufacturer of your pacemaker, which frequently has useful help pages for patients.

Appendix A

When to treat hypertension and hypercholesterolaemia

Blood pressure thresholds to initiate specific treatment

BP values (mmHg)	Joint British Societies Guidelines	American Heart Association Guidelines
130–140/80–90	*If associated with*: DM, chronic renal failure, established CV disease	*If associated with*: DM, chronic renal failure, established CV disease
140–160/90–100	*If associated with*: DM, >20% CV risk/10 years, established CV disease, target organ damage	Yes
>160/100	YES	Yes

Cholesterol levels to initiate specific treatment after a trial of diet and life-style changes*

Joint British Societies Guidelines	American Heart Association Guidelines

◆ TC >4 mmol/litre and:
  • established CV disease
  • DM
  • CV risk >20%/10 years
◆ TC/HDL-C >6
◆ Familial dyslipidaemia
	◆ LDL-C >190 mg% (5 mmol/litre) and:
	  • ≤1 other RF
	◆ LDL-C >160mg% (4 mmol/litre) and:
	  • ≥2 other RF and CV risk <10%/10 years
	◆ LDL-C > 130 mg% (3 mmol/litre)and:
	  • Σ2 other RF and CV risk >10%/10 years

CV, cardiovascular; DM, diabetes; LDL-C, LDL-cholesterol; HDL-C, HDL-cholesterol; RF, risk factor; TC, total cholesterol.

*UK guidelines focus on total cholesterol and its ratio to HDL-C as the first triage line, while US guidelines focus on LDL-C. Both sets of guidelines acknowledge the need to obtain a full lipid profile for further risk stratification.

Appendix B

Some practical advice for the cardiac patient

Before travelling abroad

◆ Consult your GP or cardiologist as to whether there is any specific aspect of your cardiac condition that you should be concerned about when travelling, especially if you have not been well of late, or there has been a change in your medication, or you are waiting for a test.

◆ Ask your GP to provide you with a short letter describing your condition, or at least a list of your diagnoses.

◆ If you have a 'rich' cardiac history or if you know you have an abnormal ECG, ask to be given a copy of it.

◆ Have a list of your medications with you and a good supply of tablets so that you will be covered for the duration of the trip.

◆ If you have a pacemaker, make sure that you take your pacemaker card with you and inform the security personnel manning detection equipment at airports.

◆ Make sure that your travel health insurance covers your existing cardiac disease, and that you are familiar with the procedure for contacting your insurance company in an emergency. This is important, especially if you travel outside the European Union.

When referred to a cardiologist in an outpatient clinic

◆ If this your first visit, or if it has been a long time since your last one, make sure that you can provide all relevant information, especially dates and details of previous admissions and interventions, if any.

◆ If you have been seen in clinic in the past, it is a good idea to ask your GP to refer you to the same hospital and cardiologist, if this is practical.

◆ Bring a list of your current medications (you do not have to bring the tablets or the vials themselves).

◆ Describe your symptoms, using your own words; avoid offering your own diagnosis. For example, if you have sudden palpitations and breathlessness, just explain what you feel. Do not say that you have 'panic attacks': this is a diagnosis in itself, and you may or may not be right, assuming that this is the problem. Also do not assume that all your problems are necessarily detailed in the referral letter, and therefore you do not have to explain what troubles you.

- Bring with you a list of questions that you would like to ask.

- If you have to be seen with results of tests, and you receive the appointment letter before the tests are performed, contact the outpatient clinic office and ask for a later appointment.

- If you have been informed that you should have a test or be seen again in clinic, and a reasonable time passes without receiving any appointment, contact the clinic office or your doctor's secretary and enquire about it.

Appendix C

Other sources of information and support

There is an increased trend for cardiac patients and their relatives to actively search for information about cardiovascular diseases, prevention, and healthy lifestyle. This 'proactive' approach has to do with mass campaigns to raise awareness of cardiac conditions, the existence of numerous patients' associations and support groups, and the easy accessibility to required information allowed by the use of the internet. Most cardiological professional bodies and many large hospitals have sections dedicated to patients on their websites. A list of suggested internet sites and organizations providing useful information for cardiac patients is provided below, although without any specific endorsement of any site. Most of them offer downloadable materials and contact details if further information is sought.

- www.nhs.uk
  - The home page of the **National Health Service** website provides two links, 'Check your health now' and 'Health A–Z', offering a wealth of information and advice on various diseases.
- www.bhf.org.uk
  - The **British Heart Foundation (BHF)** website provides updated information and advice on practically all cardiovascular conditions, heart functioning, interventions, and treatment. Both summarizing leaflets and more in-depth brochures are available to be read online, downloaded, or ordered as reprints.
- www.cardiomyopathy.org
  - The **Cardiomyopathy Association (CMA)** is a charity for the benefit of patients with cardiomyopathies and their families. They work together with the Specialist Inherited Cardiovascular Disease Clinic at the Heart Hospital in London and are recognized by the British Heart Foundation and the British Cardiovascular Society. The CMA website provides online information and allows ordering of their main booklets.
- www.heartrhythmcharity.org.uk
  - The **Arrhythmia Alliance** charity is dedicated to patients with a variety of heart rhythm disturbances. Their website has a Frequently Asked

Questions subpage and offers downloadable booklets on arrhythmias and their treatment.

◆ www.americanheart.org

    ◆ The **American Heart Association** is a major cardiological professional body in the USA. Their website homepage has a 'For patients' link opening a subpage which provides easily accessible information on risk factors and various cardiovascular conditions and their management.

◆ www.circ.ahajournals.org

    ◆ *Circulation* is one of the most prestigious cardiology journals in the USA. Under 'Browse by special section' they have a 'Cardiology Patient Page' link which offers numerous articles on cardiovascular subjects, written with the patient in mind. Many of these are downloadable free of charge.

Practical advice: by just typing a keyword of interest in your search engine, eventually with search terms as 'association', 'patient', 'advice', or 'information', you are very likely to have a large number of 'hits'. As a general caution, websites of major well-known organizations should be used to ensure that the information provided is reliable and updated.

Glossary

Aneurysm: localized dilatation of a blood vessel or of a heart cavity

Angiography (angiogram): visualization of the arteries by injecting a dye delivered by a catheter

Aorta: the largest artery in the body. It originates in the left ventricle and provides arterial branches for the whole body

Aortic valve: the valve controlling the blood flow from the ventricle to the aorta

Arrhythmia: a disorder of the heart rhythm

Atheroma: a mass of fat accumulating on the internal walls of vessels

Atherosclerosis: hardening and narrowing of the arteries due to fat build-up on their walls

Atria: the two upper cavities of the heart (singular: atrium)

Bradycardia: slow heart rate

Capillaries: small (5–10 microns in diameter) thin-walled vessels that connect the endings of the arteries and of the veins, surround and penetrate tissues, and allow the circulation of blood to and from the cells

Cardiomyopathy: a disease of the heart muscle

Cardiac: related to the heart

Cardiovascular: related to the heart and vessels

Carotid arteries: the two main neck arteries

Caval veins: two large veins (superior and inferior vena cava) that collect the venous blood from the whole body and return it to the right atrium

Cerebral: related to the brain

Coronary arteries: the arteries that provide blood to the heart itself

Cranial: related to the skull

Diastole: phase of cardiac cycle when the ventricles relax and increase their dimensions to fill with blood

Diuretic: a drug promoting urine formation

Dyspnoea: breathlessness

Echocardiography: high-quality non-invasive imaging of the heart using ultrasound technology

Electrocardiogram: recording of the electrical activity of the heart, obtained by connecting the patient's arms and chest to a specialized machine

Embolus: a piece of material (generally a clot) that travels with the blood and can lodged in vessel

Endocarditis: inflammation or infection of the inner layer of the heart

Endocardium: the inner layer of the heart

Fibrillation: a rapid and disorganized electrical or mechanical activity

Flutter: a rapid but regular electrical activity

Heart attack: lay term for myocardial infarction. Not to be used for any other acute heart condition

Hepatic: related to the liver

Hormone: a substance synthesized by a gland, such as the thyroid, and released into blood to control the function of other organs or tissues

Hypertrophy: increased thickness or mass of a tissue due to increase in the size of cells

Infarction: death of cells due to lack of blood supply

Ischaemia: a condition whereby tissue and organs are deprived of oxygen because of decreased blood supply

Leaflet: leaf-like valvular structure whose motion opens or closes the valve

Lipids: general name for fats

Lumen: the internal free space through which a fluid or a gas can move in a conduit

Metabolism: cycle of chemical reactions occurring in living cells, ensuring that they grow and perform their functions. Metabolism has two components: catabolism, relating to breaking down of nutrients to generate energy, and anabolism, relating to building and synthesis of cell components

Mitral valve: valve made from two leaflets that controls the blood flow from the left atrium to the left ventricle

Myocardium: the heart muscle

Oedema: swelling of soft tissues

Paroxysmal: occurring suddenly and ceasing spontaneously

Pericardium: the outer layer of the heart

Prophylaxis: prevention

Pulmonary: related to the lungs

Renal: related to the kidneys

Saturated fats: fats whose molecules have all the available positions filled by hydrogen. Fats that are solid at room temperature are generally saturated and may raise cholesterol levels (bad fats)

Septum: a wall separating internal cavities

Stenosis: narrowing

Syncope: sudden fainting with loss of consciousness

Systole: phase of cardiac cycle when the ventricles contract

Tachycardia: rapid heart rate

Transudation: a process of passage of fluid through vessels walls

Thrombolytic: a drug or process that breaks a clot

Thrombus: blood clot

Tricuspid valve: a valve made from three cusps that controls the blood flow from the right atrium to the right ventricle

Unsaturated fats: fats whose molecules have more double bonds, and thus less hydrogen. Fats that are fluid at room temperature are generally unsaturated and may lower cholesterol (good fats)

Ventricles: the two lower cavities of the heart (brain cavities are also called ventricles)

Index

Index entries appear in word-by-word alphabetical order.